Keto Vegan

A beginner guide to plant-based and Ketogenic diet, live a healthy lifestyle and reach the best from your body

[Dr Steven Green]

Legal & Disclaimer

You agree to accept all risks of using the information presented inside this book.

You agree that by continuing to read this book, where appropriate and/or necessary, you shall consult a professional (including but not limited to your doctor, attorney, or financial advisor or such other advisor as needed) before using any of the suggested remedies, techniques, or information in this book.

Table of Contents

INTRODUCTION

Ketogenic diet is a low-carb diet that helps your body burn fat effectively. This attribute is derived from the fact that a keto diet induces your body to produce minute fuel molecules known as "ketones", which are alternative energy sources for the body.

Your body produces these molecules when your blood sugar is in short supply, and this can only happen if you consume just a few carbs with each meal When following a ketogenic diet, your body switches to consuming the body's fat for energy, which is one of the basics when you are trying to lose weight.

Other less obvious benefits of the keto diet include feeling less hungry and having higher energy levels, all of which contribute to keeping your body alert and focused.

How the ketogenic diet works?

In the ketogenic diet, a natural mechanism of the body is exploited. Carbohydrates, which the body does not need immediately, are converted into fat and stored. This releases insulin, which also prevents the burning of fat. By abstaining from carbohydrates in the diet, fat burning is stimulated. The body is put into hunger metabolism, ketosis. The reduction of carbohydrates promotes fat burning. The amount of carbohydrates that can be consumed at the most varies - about 30 g of carbohydrates is the maximum amount to achieve hunger metabolism. For example, not more than 40 g of pasta may be eaten per day. This is problematic insofar as the German Nutrition Society recommends eating at least 200 g of carbohydrates with a calorie requirement of 2,000 calories. Instead of providing the body with calories from carbohydrates, many proteins come from meat, dairy, and eggs. This is to prevent the loss of muscle when losing weight.

Chapter 1: What is Plant-Based diet

In simple terms, a plant-based diet means consuming food that comes from plants. A plant-based diet does not include ingredients that come from animals, such as milk, meat, honey, or eggs. With a plant-based diet, it is now possible to meet your nutritional requirements with only natural and minimally processed items.

A plant-based diet includes fruits, vegetables, and tubers. A diet laden with veggies, fruits, tubers, and whole grains will help you diminish the harmful effects of many chronic diseases. For instance, did you know that a diet full of fresh fruits and veggies can lower blood pressure and control Type 2 diabetes?

You need not feel apprehensive about this change, because going for a plant-based diet does not necessarily mean that you will turn vegan. Neither do you have to give up on dairy or meat. It is rather an informed decision to primarily choose food items sourced from plants.

Plant-based diets like the Mediterranean diet have been proven to reduce the risk of certain cancers, metabolic disorders, and even heart disease. In older adults, a plant-based diet has also been effective in reducing the effects of depression and increasing physical and mental function.

The plant-based diet seems confusing due to many arguments that describe it to be either a vegan or vegetarian diet. There are also claims that suggest that the plant-based diet should include some amount of animal products or none at all.

In reality, no studies have concretely defined what the plant-based diet is, which leaves this lifestyle up to the dieter's discretion.

The plant-based diet is merely a style of eating that focuses on having plant foods as a major part of each meal. It could be a 100% plant-food style or could have more plant-foods merged with little amounts of animal-foods.

For this reason, one may suggest that the plant-based diet is either a vegan diet (with 100% plant food focus) or a vegetarian diet (with the use of some animal products). Both cases are overruled, and I will tell you why.

Aside from the plant-based diet constructing its foods from plants, it intensely rejects processed foods like bleached rice and added sugars. However, the vegan and vegetarian diets allow some amounts of processed foods, which would disqualify them from being called the plant-based diet.

The choice of managing plant to animal to processed foods on the plant-based diet relies on the dieter's discretion, eating habits, and health goals. For this reason, I will prefer not to justify a course for how such proportions should be managed.

What to eat on the WFPB?

Now that I talk of plant-focused foods, let's count the many options that you can enjoy.

- Fruits

All fruits are permitted on the plant-based diet and they can be enjoyed either fresh, frozen, or sun-dried. Eat the wide range of citrus fruits, berries, grapes, apples, melons, bananas, peaches, apricots, avocado, kiwi fruits, etc.

- Vegetables

A healthful plant-based sits in a wide range of vegetables. All vegetables are welcomed on the diet both above the ground and under the ground vegetables. Meanwhile, vegetables provide a wide range of vitamins and minerals.

Enjoy spinach, kale, mustard greens, collard greens, broccoli, cauliflower, asparagus, green beans, eggplants, carrots, tomatoes, bell peppers, zucchinis, beetroot, parsnips, turnips, potatoes, etc.

- Legumes

Legumes are an excellent source for plant-based protein and fiber. Fiber is one nutrient that many people lack; hence, it is necessary to consume foods like legumes often to enrich the body with enough fiber.

Eat the wide range of beans, chickpeas, lentils, peas, etc.

- Whole Grains

These are also fantastic for fiber sourcing and help maintain stable blood sugar. They are also rich in essential minerals like selenium, copper, and magnesium.

It is important to note that whole grains vary from bleached grains, therefore avoid processed flours, rice, pasta, and breads on the plant-based diet.

Eat brown rice, whole-wheat pasta, whole-grain bread, oats, barley, buckwheat, rye, quinoa, spelt, corn, etc.

- Nuts and Nut Butters

Nuts are an essential source of selenium, vitamin E, and plant-based protein. They are excellent additions to smoothies, puddings, desserts, and snacks.

Crunch on almonds, pecans, walnuts, macadamia nuts, hazelnuts, pistachios, cashew nuts, peanuts, brazil, etc.

- Seeds

Incorporate seeds into soups, snacks, smoothies, desserts, etc. They are rich in calcium, Vitamin E, and are a good source of healthy fats.

Consume flaxseeds, pepitas (pumpkin seeds), sunflower seeds, chia seeds, hemp seeds, sesame seeds, etc.

- Healthy Oils and Fats

Fats do not have to come from animal sources only. Some plant foods equally provide excellent fats for frying, searing, baking, and act as replacement for most dairy products. Meanwhile, they are rich in omega-3 fatty acids.

Use olive oil, avocados, canola oil, walnuts, peanuts, hemp seeds, flaxseeds, chia seeds, cashew nuts, coconut oil, etc.

- Plant-Based Milk, Cream, and Cheeses

Going plant-based doesn't mean starving yourself off creamy, milky, cheesy foods. You can enjoy plant-based alternatives of pasta alfredo, cheesecakes, etc.

Enjoy almond milk, soy milk, coconut milk, coconut cream, rice milk, cashew milk, cashew cream, hemp milk, oats milk, etc.

- Plant-Based Meats

Also, enrich your foods with meats options made from plant sources like soymilk and whole grains.

Eat tofu, tempeh, seitan, etc.

- Spices, Herbs, and Condiments

Nothing beats the preparation of foods than the aroma that exudes while cooking. Therefore, all ranges of homemade spices, herbs, and condiments are welcomed.

Use basil, parsley, rosemary, oregano, thyme, sage, marjoram, turmeric, curry, black pepper, salt, salsa, soy sauce, nutritional yeast, vinegar, homemade BBQ sauce, homemade plant-based mayonnaise, etc.

- Beverages

Coffee, sparking water, tea, smoothies, etc. are fine to drink.

Foods to avoid on the WFPB

For sticking to whole-foods on the plant-based diet, it is essential to eliminate animal products entirely. Also, avoid eating the following foods:

- Processed foods – prefer to use homemade unprocessed versions.

- Excess salt – many salt brands are highly processed while excess salt intake increases high blood pressure. Reduce your salt intake.

- Refined white carbohydrates – like white rice, white bread, white pasta.

- Sugary foods – swap them for fresh fruits, smoothies, freshly squeezed juices, etc. Avoid store-bought cakes, biscuits, pastries, soda, artificially flavored drinks, etc.

- Processed vegan and vegetarian alternatives that may include high amounts of salt and sugar.

- Greasy, fatty, and deep-fried foods – work with little amounts of fats as much as possible.

Sourcing vital nutrients on the WFPB

While the plant-based lifestyle comes with numerous benefits, not focusing on deriving other essential nutrients that will mostly be found in animal-foods can be harmful to your health. Instead, source these nutrients from the following:

- Vitamin B-12

Vitamin B-12 is a crucial nutrient for cell and blood health. A deficiency in this nutrient can lead to nerve damage and anemia. Therefore, dieters can consider taking B-12 supplements or eat foods like plant-based milk, whole-wheat cereals, and nutritional yeast.

- Protein

Thankfully, many whole grains and vegetables are an excellent source for protein. There isn't a need to worry about losing out on protein on the WFPB. Source protein from tofu, quinoa, chickpeas, beans, nuts, seeds, and mushrooms.

- Iron

Iron requires a bit of intentional seeking when on the diet. This requirement is because iron has a lower bioavailability in plants and meats. Therefore, dieters should incorporate these foods into their meals at least two to three times weekly. Eat cabbage, soybeans, black beans, kidney beans, raisins, cashews, oatmeal, tomato juice, spinach, and dark leafy greens.

To increase iron absorption, ensure to combine citrus and other vitamin C sources with these plant-based foods.

- Omega-3 Fatty Acids

Omega-3 fatty acids are essential for reducing inflammation, memory, and other chronic conditions. However, they are highly sourced from fish, seafood, and other animal sources.

To derive your fair share of this nutrient from plant foods, consume hempseeds, walnuts, and flaxseeds. However, at digestion the body derives omega-3 ALA, which the body finds slow to convert to EPA and DHA, the two-primary omega-3 fatty acids that the body can use immediately.

Therefore, for WFPB dieters, it is essential to substitute with plant-based omega-3 fatty acids supplements.

Chapter 2: Benefits of Plant-Based diet

A plant-based diet helps improve your gut health. Items sourced from plants are full of rich fiber, and this improves digestion. Fiber will add bulk to stool and regulate the entire digestive process.

As plants are rich in minerals and vitamins, they are great energy boosters. You will find them full of phytonutrients, antioxidants, and healthy protein and fat. All these are good for both the body and the brain. Plant-sourced items are easier to digest, which helps the body by giving it some extra energy.

Plant-based diets are known to reverse the effects of chronic diseases like cancer, heart disease, and diabetes. People who have shifted to a plant-based diet are at a lower risk for chronic diseases like heart disease, diabetes, and even Alzheimer's.

A plant-based diet can also help give you glowing skin and healthy nails. As the food items are full of minerals and vitamins, they are perfect for your skin.

If you are trying to lose weight, it's time to bring some change with a plant-based diet. These nutrient-dense food items can help you lose weight effectively, as you consume a fewer calories naturally by following a plant-based diet.

Of course, if you are an animal lover, having a plant-based diet will be awesome. You are getting your nutrition from nature without harming any animals.

Chapter 3: What is Ketogenic diet

In addition, the fat content is increased. This should cause the body does not continue to store fat because it does not fear that too little fat is available. The ingredients are chosen in the ketogenic diet so that 70-80% of fat is available. 20-25% of the diet is said to be protein, while at most 5% is carbohydrate. Other approaches incorporate more carbohydrates into the diet, so the proportion is up to 20%. The fat content is then reduced to 70% and the protein content to 10%. The fats are chosen to achieve weight loss in such moderate variants so that they form more ketone bodies. This is achieved by medium-chain fatty acids, which are present in coconut oil.

<u>Benefits of keto diet</u> .

Type 2 diabetes

The carbohydrate limitation can have a direct effect on glucose concentration and reduce it over time. It can be a simple way to control your diabetes

But you should consult a registered dietitian before applying this strategy. As a general, a healthy diet and carbohydrate control can give the same results.

Cancer

This is a growing field of research for the keto diet. The Warburg effect has shown that tumor cells can break down glucose much faster (200x faster) than typical cells. The theory is that starving tumor cells from glucose can inhibit their growth and prevent cancer.

Keto is ideal for a predominantly sedentary lifestyle

Sedentary lifestyles are too common - a lifestyle often dictated by desk jobs and long hours. Even if you exercise for about 30 minutes in a day and the rest of the day are rather inactive, there are good reasons to keep carbohydrate intake low because you do not need muscle glycogen.

In addition, you can make the carbohydrates you have work more efficiently for you by scheduling your intake around your pre-workout and post-workout plan.

A period of low carbohydrate intake via the ketogenic diet can help to increase your sensitivity to insulin and ensure that you can reintroduce carbohydrates at a later time, without cost for physique or performance.

We can consider as benefits:

1) Accelerated fat burning

Avoiding sugar Carbohydrates is one of the most effective ways to lose as much fat and, thus, excess body weight in a short time.

The reason is that low-carb diets in the first step remove excess water from your body, then lower your insulin levels and ultimately reduce your hunger/appetite.

In the long run, ketosis transforms your body into a fat-burning machine that operates 24 hours a day, 7 days a week.

2) Stable and low blood sugar level

Millions of people all over the world suffer from diabetes or high insulin resistance. The best thing for these people is that the ketogenic diet can provide some benefits.

Avoiding carbohydrates can dramatically decrease your blood sugar levels, preventing fatigue or starvation.

3) Increased stamina

Even endurance athletes can boost their performance through ketosis. This is because energy production from ketones and fatty acids consumes less oxygen and is generally more efficient.

The FASTER study is one of the best-known and large-scale studies in this field. The researchers studied the effects of ketosis on the endurance of athletes - with amazing results.

In summary, the keto athletes differed by more powerful mitochondria, accelerated fat burning, less oxygen demand, and a slightly increased efficiency.

4) Better sleep quality

Sleep and especially deep sleep has been proven to be one of the most important processes in our body. Again, ketosis can work wonders!

This is because ketosis activates cell-internal "garbage collection" on the one hand and the other hand, leads to efficient energy production. Therefore report Ketarier often of a better quality of sleep and a decrease in the need for sleep.

5) Improved brain functions

Another well-researched advantage of the ketogenic diet is the enhancement of brain functions such as memory, concentration, or focus.

Several human studies have confirmed the beneficial effects of ketosis on the memory of adults.

Besides, ketosis leads to an increase in the production of mitochondria in the human brain, which can increase the concentration of ATP in the brain, and especially in your hippocampus.

6) Higher metabolic rate and energy consumption

basal metabolic rate is the amount of energy your body requires per day to keep the most important functions going in your body.

Some studies have linked low carb or ketogenic diet to higher basal metabolic rates. This means that weight can be lost faster in the long term or define the body or muscles.

7) Nutrient-rich diet

Foods that should eat in the ketogenic diet include fish, vegetables, high-quality meat, and other unrefined foods.

These foods are rich in minerals and required nutrients that contribute to the health and performance of your body.

8) Lower blood pressure

Just as exciting: hypertensive patients can benefit from a ketogenic diet.

It is confirmed that a low-carb diet and forms of the ketogenic diet can reduce some important risk factors of various heart diseases. This includes lower blood pressure.

9) Stronger mitochondria

Mitochondria are the cell power plants of our bodies. Without them, the energy would go out within a few minutes. Most of our health, performance, and immune system rely on the function of our mitochondria.

In general, one can conclude from their research that ketosis can measurably increase the performance and number of mitochondria in the body.

10) Slower aging process

One way to mitigate the aging of the body is to reduce oxidative stress. Interestingly, low insulin levels lead to less oxidative stress.

Avoiding sugar and other carbohydrates as part of a ketogenic diet will sustainably lower the blood sugar and insulin levels in the body, which in turn will measurably and noticeably slow down your aging process.

11) Faster and stronger satiety

Many diets cause one thing above all else: a constant feeling of hunger. The keto diet is different here - because it can be proven to lead to a stronger feeling of satiety, which also occurs even faster.

Several studies show that carbohydrate-wasting and consumption of more fat and protein results in less hunger and a lower calorie count every year.

This will allow you to burn fat in less time - without the unpleasant feeling of constant and ubiquitous hunger!

12) Fasting becomes much easier

Everyone knows the feeling when we give up our lunch or forgot about dinner because of hard work.

As part of a normal diet, most people find it hard to forego any food for 12 hours even though fasting can have incredible health benefits. It's different in ketosis: it's no longer a problem if you do not eat for 12,

16, or even 24 hours. As a result, prolonged or intermittent fasting (16-hour daily fasting) will be much easier.

13) Better mood & mood

There are many effects of the ketogenic diet on people with autism.

Among other things, this effect is due to the increased formation of GABA and serotonin in the course of ketosis. The distribution of these happy hormones, in turn, means that Ketarier often reports an improved mood.

Another convincing reason to forego sugar and simple carbohydrates in the future!

14) Faster weight loss

It has been scientifically proven that low carb and high-fat diets are the most efficient way to lose plenty of weight and fat in a short period of time.

On the one hand, this is because to much water (which is bound to carbohydrates and glycogen) is excreted.

Second, you turn your body into an efficient fat-burning machine. In this way, you will burn fat faster and more effectively over the long term and lose weight.

15) Higher HDL cholesterol

HDL cholesterol (high-density lipoprotein) is also often referred to the good cholesterol. The higher the amount of HDL, relative to the "bad" LDL, the lower the risk of heart disease.

Through the high consumption of healthy fatty acids in the course of the ketogenic diet, you can raise the amount of "good" HDL cholesterol and thus prevent heart disease.

16) Increased libido

Ketosis can significantly increase the quality of life of men through increased testosterone levels and more libidos.

This effect gets stronger the more high-quality fats (MCT, coconut fat, etc.) you eat like a man in ketosis.

17) Lower insulin levels

Low-carb diets and ketogenic nutrition are particularly beneficial for people with diabetes and high insulin resistance - these conditions affect several million people worldwide.

Studies have shown that people suffering from diabetes can reduce their insulin levels up to 50 percent with a low / no-carb diet.

18) Faster getting up in the morning

Because of the improved sleep quality we wrote earlier in the article, many Ketarians report more energy and willpower to get them out of bed in the morning.

19) Improved LDL cholesterol level

People with too high an LDL level are more likely to have a heart attack during their lifetime.

In ketosis, the size of LDL particles rises, while the absolute number of particles mitigates. As the LDL particles become larger, the lower the risk of myocardial infarction.

Therefore, by avoiding sugar and carbohydrates, you can reduce the risk of a heart attack!

20) Reduces symptoms of allergies

In addition, ketosis balances and soothes the human immune system. Since an allergy is nothing but an overreaction of the immune system, ketosis can reduce the symptoms of allergies.

21) Ketose has an anticatabolic effect

Especially athletes are afraid to lose hard-earned muscle mass in ketosis

Ketones have an anticatabolic effect in your body. This means that the signal to your body that it should not reduce muscle but fat.

DISADVANTAGES OF KETOGENIC DIET

Difficult to hold out

Ketosis is difficult to achieve because it is like a light switch: either on or off. People who consistently follow food intake tend to stay in ketosis. But the best way to tell if your body is in ketosis is a blood test.

Nutrient deficiency

Each food group offers a different essential diet. Focus on meat, seafood, vegetables, some legumes, and fruits to make sure you get fiber, B vitamins, and minerals like iron, magnesium, and zinc. It would be best to consult with a registered nutritionist to reduce the possibility of deficiencies.

Keto flu

During the diet transition, you may experience unpleasant side effects of significantly reduced carbohydrates, sometimes referred to as "keto flu." Hunger, headache, nausea, fatigue, irritability, constipation, and "fog" in the brain can take days. Sleep and hydration help, but it can not be a smooth transition to nutrition.

Bad fats in practice

The high-fat content of the diet could have a negative impact on heart health. The American Heart Association recommends limiting the intake of saturated fat to 5 to 6 percent. "In practice, many people eat high levels of saturated fats, which could increase the risk of cardiovascular disease,"

Renal risk

"Patients with kidney disease are at a higher risk of dialysis on the keto diet because their kidney system needs to handle additional ketones," says Dr. Maganti.

Some people also experience dehydration on the ketone diet because they eliminate glycogen, which keeps water out of their bloodstream.

Food obsession

"Micromanaging your food intake by tracking how much you eat separates you from what your body demands," says Gomez. "You start using external numbers to decide what to eat instead of listening to your body."

Such close monitoring of food can lead to psychological problems such as shame and intoxication. Restriction can lead to intoxication, which often leads to feelings of guilt, which then leads to a restriction in a continuous cycle.

Chapter 4: Different types of Dieting

There are so many diet patterns these days, and it's hard to maintain them. Do it for reasons of health, environmental protection, or animal rights.

Paleo:

The paleo diet is simple. It's a diet for cabbage people, which means you do not eat processed foods or anything that has not been on the ground. Why did people become paleo? Well, if cabbage people eat essential foods like meat and poultry that eat grass, fish, eggs, vegetables, natural oils, fruits, nuts, and cereals are lean, muscular and sports, why not eat like them?

Vegan:

No animals were damaged in this type of food. Vegan, without any animals or by-products such as meat, fish, dairy products, honey, and eggs, eat herbal foods containing alternative proteins, fake cheeses, and fruits and vegetables. Increasingly affordable for cruelty to animals and environmental reasons, products abound in the vegan market, such as counterfeit meat, dairy-free yogurt, alternative cheese, etc.

Variations:

Vegan Keto: Without meat and dairy products, very little bread, and pasta, but a lot of vegetation.

Paleo Keto: This protein is fed with grass, fish, eggs, vegetables, and fruits. Say hello to all the processed carbs.

Foods

They can all agree on: If you have friends and one is vegan, one is fading, and the other is keto, this may seem like the worst gastronomic nightmare in the history of accommodation. Do not panic (tap). Salads are of course the most comfortable option because everyone can eat salads and other vegetables, as well as essential oils such as olive oil. Other options include rice in bloom, stuffed avocado, zoodles with creamy sauce or rice flour and mushroom puree. Sounds pretty good, does not it?

Chapter 5: What is the difference between Ketosis and Vegan

Ketosis is a natural stage of the body in which the body produces its energy through the consumption of fat. The name ketosis comes from the fact that your liver in this state produces small molecules, called ketone bodies, from the conversion of fatty acids.

Usually, glucose in the form of sugar or carbohydrates is the primary energy source of our body. If we do not receive glucose replenishment for more than 24 to 48 hours, fatty acids and ketone bodies are used for cellular energy production.

Vegan diets provide other critically essential nutrients such as Vitamins E and C, phytochemicals, antioxidants, and foliate. These help in keeping your immunity system healthy and robust, and also prevent age-related diseases such as Alzheimer's and Parkinson's disease and keep your overall body organs functioning well.

Vegan diets have the power to prevent the following diseases that are very common in today's high-stress unhealthy lifestyle:

- Cardiovascular diseases

- Reduced cholesterol due to the complete absence of meat and dairy products in your diet

- Age-related macular degeneration

- Reduced risk of breast cancer

- Reduced risk of contracting ailments like diabetes, hypertension, cataracts, colon and prostate cancer, arthritis, and osteoporosis

In addition to improved health and prevention of diseases, going vegan makes you stronger, more energetic, and more attractive. Here is how:

Lowered Body Mass Index – Cutting meat and dairy out of your diet naturally reduces Body Mass Index.

Weight loss – Weight loss is an unquestioned effect of a vegan diet.

Healthy skin – Consuming rich sources of Vitamins A and E from nuts and fruits and vegetables enhance the texture and health of your skin.

Reduced allergy symptoms – Plant-based foods do not trigger as many allergic reactions in humans as dairy and meat products do.

Less intake of mercury – A lot of shellfish and fish contain high levels of mercury, which we take in when we eat these foods. Switching to veganism does away with this toxin completely.

The above are only some of the great reasons that you must start off this 30-day vegan challenge. Instead of finding reasons not to do something good, focus on the above reasons which tell you why you should do it and dive straight in. Summon some extra willpower and after you complete this challenge you can rest assured that the willpower would come on its own when you see and feel the wondrous new VEGAN YOU.

Chapter 6: What is Vegan Lifestyle

Most people in the world want to do the following things by some means or the other:

- Lose weight

- Eat better

- Get fitter and healthier

- Do something for society and the world at large

The great news is that if you shift to a vegan diet, you can achieve all the above goals. And let me assure you, you will enjoy delicious, wholesome, and satiating meals as well.

No loss or reduction in energy levels – There is a misconception that changing to a vegan diet reduces your energy levels. There are numerous unworthy talks of vegans living only on water and a few greens and hence their energy levels have taken a huge dip. And on the other side of the spectrum, there are plenty of spurious rumors that say going vegan is helping them do impossible things. These other-end-of-the-spectrum talks make out vegans to be people who can walk on water! Let me assure you that neither of the extremes is true or based on any scientific studies.

Health benefits are huge when you choose to go vegan. Of course, the initial learning curve is going to be steep and you would have to counter multiple challenges. However, once you have overcome these tough phases and complete the 30-day challenge, you are going feel to happier, lighter, and fit. Moreover, there are multiple studies done by various organizations including the British Dietetic Association that has proven the excellent efficacies of getting fitter and healthier by following a vegan diet.

Here is the list of a few magic foods that can restore energy instantaneously:

Bananas – Already beautifully and naturally packaged by nature, this wonderful tropical fruit is normally the first you must reach out for when you feel tired or fatigued.

Walnuts – Another great pick-me-up tree nut, walnuts are rich in plant proteins, omega fatty acids, and vitamins giving you the almost-instant energy boost.

Green smoothies – Delicious smoothies made by tossing together strawberries, bananas, and orange juices are great and extremely healthy pick-me-ups to fight fatigue.

Coconut water – This is nature's energy drink and is amazingly refreshing and is filled with vitamins and potassium.

Kiwi – This low-fat delicious fruit is an instant energy enhancer triggered by the simple sugars present in it.

Why I chose to mention vegan energy boosters in the beginning itself is to help you overcome doubts regarding your ability to get on with your daily schedule if you choose to go vegan. Today there are many sportspeople who have shifted to this diet to keep fitter and sustain energy levels. So, if highly active people in the field of sports can take advantage of veganism, it should not be difficult for moderately active people like us to take this 30-day challenge and come out with flying colors.

Other great reasons to take the one-month challenge to go vegan are:

Lose weight and yet remain energized – Many of us would love to find a sensible way to lose excess weight and yet remain healthy and fit. Average vegans are known to weigh 20 pounds lesser than average meat-eaters. Despite this, vegan diets do not starve you and make you feel enervated like the usual run-of-the-meal fad diets do.

Keep diseases and health disorders away – The Academy of Nutrition and Dietetics have conducted multiple studies which show that taking the vegan route helps you steer clear of common disorders such as diabetes, hypertension or high blood pressure thereby preventing the onset of many modern-day diseases such as heart attacks, kidney failure, and others.

Vegan foods are yummy and delicious – If you thought going vegan means you would have to give up your favorite ice creams, hamburgers, and chicken sandwiches, then you are wrong. With demand for vegan products soaring, many companies are coming up with amazingly delicious vegan options that taste very much like the non-vegetarian stuff. You will not miss any of the meats and animal products at all. There are plenty of established brands that cater to veganism and deliver really tasty dairy and meat substitutes.

Vegan diets are full of highly nutritious and healthy food items including whole grains, beans and legumes, nuts, soy products, and fresh fruits and vegetables. Here are some of the health benefits that these fiber-rich and healthy food sources provide you with:

- **Minimal saturated fats** – Meats and dairy products contain plenty of saturated fats thereby increasing the risk of cardiovascular diseases. Vegan diets automatically reduce intake of saturated fats enhancing your health condition

- **Fiber** – A vegan diet is high in fiber content that is very conducive to healthy bowel movements.

- **Magnesium** – Dark, green leafy vegetables are a rich source of magnesium, a key element that aids the body in the absorption of calcium.

- **Potassium** – Similarly, potassium, an important mineral that balances acidity and water in our body and helps in the removal of toxins, is found plenty in plant-based foods.

- **Proteins** – Meat-eaters invariably end up with more proteins than is needed by the body. Vegan diets, which include nuts, beans, and legumes, have the right amount of proteins for us.

Chapter 7: Tips and Tricks to reach your Best shape

Before you dive into a new diet, you should always make sure that you know what that diet is and what it entails. So, first things first. What is a ketogenic diet? A ketogenic diet is categorized as a diet, this being very low carb but very high fat. This is not the first time most people are hearing this as they've heard about other diets of this sort as well. While this diet can be similar to others, there are also differences that set it apart. What this diet is designed to do is it puts your body into a state called ketosis. This is a metabolic state that is a reduction of carbs and it means you're reducing how much your intake of carbs is and instead, you're replacing it with fat. They believe that when you adopt this diet, your body will become more efficient at burning your fat and turning it into energy. It's also believed that the fats in your liver will turn into ketones. After they turn to ketones, it is said by some that your brain will now have more energy because of this process.

As with a vegetarian diet, there are people who classify themselves as a different type of ketogenic. While there is a debate on which is the best, there are four that are most commonly chosen among people.

The high protein ketogenic diet, which has things in common with a standard ketogenic diet (but as the title implies), has more protein than the standard version. The ratio is, of course, different as well. For a high protein ketogenic diet, you have thirty-five percent proteins, with sixty percent fat and only five percent is made up of carbs.

The targeted ketogenic diet is another ketogenic diet that a lot of people enjoy. This one is very similar to the others except that for this, a targeted ketogenic diet allows you to add carbs to your diet around workouts. This is actually one of two ketogenic diets on this list that allows you to change the number of carbs that you're allowed to use.

A cyclical ketogenic diet is a diet that uses the idea of Refeeding is the process of eating more calories than you have in previous days. People believe that the process of refeeding is beneficial in losing fat because it is supposed to boost metabolism and ideally stop you from falling into a calorie deficit or crashing. So, this diet will be using higher refeeds than the other forms of ketogenic diets on this list. This is the only one on this list that allows you to have cheat days. They believe that you should have two higher carb days and five ketogenic days. They also stress that the two carb days should follow the ketogenic days and not before.

Finally, we come to the standard ketogenic diet. This is the most popular of the four and most people choose this diet as their go-to for this lifestyle. The standard diet believes that you should have only twenty percent protein and five percent carbs but have a seventy-five percent allowance for your fat. It is most assuredly a high-fat diet with extremely low carbs but still maintaining moderate protein. The thing to remember here is low carb. There are many vegan foods that you shouldn't eat on a ketogenic diet like pasta, tortillas, bread, pretzels and other snack foods like chips or crackers, soda, cereal, fruit juices, and most fruits. These are all too high in carbs for a ketogenic diet. You'll need to stay away from packaged foods with refined flour or sugar, rice, white potatoes, sweet potatoes, and starchy vegetables. There are still plenty of other items you can eat so if it seems like you're really limited, you're not. You just need to work around what you can't eat.

Any of these diets would benefit you although obviously, as each diet has differences, you will need to determine which is going to help you the most because you know what your goals are.

Originally, a ketogenic diet was believed to be a helpful aid to help with epilepsy and seizures. One of the things that are stressed about this is that the ketogenic diet is very specialized since it needs to be done with the guidance, supervision, and care of trained medical specialists. In certain countries of the world, they will only offer adult treatment in very few clinics because more data and research are needed about the impact the diet will have on adults. Through careful monitoring with specialists, doctors, and nutritionists, they say there can be benefits for children with epilepsy and seizures using this diet, but they are still conducting more research on this as well.

Other studies have shown that the ketogenic diet may reduce symptoms of Parkinson's disease or polycystic ovary syndrome in women by reducing insulin levels. It has been debated in others that it may be used to treat different kinds of cancer or tumor growth or reduce symptoms of Alzheimer's disease or possibly slow down its progression. When scientists did a study on animals, they learned that on an animal brain, the diet could reduce concussions and help recovery after a brain injury but obviously, an animal's brain is vastly different than humans and we don't know if the same results would be reflected in a human brain.

It has been debated but, in some cases, people found that some of the test subjects lost two times more weight on the ketogenic diet than on a low-fat diet that restricts calories. Like veganism, which means that you don't consume any animal product at all whatsoever, a ketogenic diet is also said to help with type two diabetes. However, the ketogenic diet is said in one study to have improved insulin by seventy-five percent.

Another study even found that seven people out of the twenty-one participants were able to stop using their diabetic medication. Now, obviously, that doesn't mean it will happen for everyone as everyone's health and body can be different and some people may have had diabetes longer than others. That's why more research is needed on the subject so that we can have more concrete answers and evidence.

Chapter 8: Live a HEALTHY lifestyle

A multivitamin in combination with your regular vegan diet supplements should supply you with the perfect amount of each of these smaller micronutrients. You should, however, consult your physician before you start taking iron supplements. Tracking your macronutrients is definitely more involved, but there's a special tool that we're going to borrow from the body-building community to make it easier.

How Weighing Your Portions Ensures Success

Nobody likes a scale, but isn't it true that everything's better when there's food involved? Back when the fitness community began to really focus on how our diets were facilitating weight loss, many body-builders and intense athletes started to use food scales as a way to be more precise about the portion sizes. But not just portions of whole meals—weighing your food with a food scale allows you to calculate the number of macronutrients **and** the number of calories in each portion of the meals you're going to prepare each week. The first step to using your food scale is to download an app called MyFitnessPal (the most popular macronutrient tracking app out there, and a great community to get involved with if you're vegan!). If you don't have a smartphone, feel free to use an online calculator—you'll be able to find more than a few. The next step is to visit your local restaurant supply store to stock up on large containers. Each week, when you prepare your meal on Sunday, you'll want to use your food scale to weight the entire cooked meal (all three or four portions together). To do this, set your chosen container on your scale and make the numbers read "00.00" – you're going to be pouring your entire meal into these containers to measure, so bigger is better. Once you've measured the full meal, use your application to plug in each of the ingredients you used in the meal and their amounts. This is just another reason that it's important to be organized with your grocery shopping. The resulting numbers should give you the number of total calories and nutrients, and if you divide by the number of portions you intend for the meal to make, you'll have an accurate nutritional label of calories, vitamins, and nutrients.

Chapter 9: What to Eat and What to Avoid

FOODS TO EAT

1. Vegetables

Vegetables contain essential fiber, vitamins, minerals, and phytochemicals. Therefore, it has a high priority in a healthy diet and is vital for our digestive system.

Allowed vegetables:

Spinach, cucumber, broccoli, cauliflower, zucchini, Brussels sprouts, Chinese cabbage, fennel, kale, celeriac, radishes, asparagus, savoy cabbage, asparagus, avocado, bitter green, bok choi, cauliflower, cabbage, celery, chard, cabbage, endive, kohlrabi, lettuce , Nori, olives, radishes, summer squash, artichoke

Recommendation: In a ketogenic diet, you should focus on low-starch vegetables. However, there is nothing wrong with eating sweet potato, pumpkin, or beetroot now and then.

2. Healthy fat

Healthy fat is the primary source of energy in a ketogenic diet. Approximately 70-80% of all calories should come from this category.

Allowed fat:

Coconut oil, olive oil, avocado oil, MCT oil, caprylic acid, fish oil, krill oil, cod liver oil, willow butter, grape ghee, sunflower lecithin, almond paste, cocoa butter, lard from grazing (unhardened), egg yolk

Recommendation: Consume at least two tablespoons of MCT oil or pure caprylic acid daily. The body converts the medium-chain fatty acids contained into three metabolic steps.

3. High-quality proteins

For a properly conducted ketogenic diet, one should not exaggerate the protein consumption. Find out more in the article " Ketogenic nutrition: benefits and implementation at a glance."

Allowed foods:

Free-range eggs, fat wild-caught fish, grazing pasture, game, grape-based collagen hydrolyzate, whey protein from grazing, vegetable protein powder

Recommendation: Do not overdo protein consumption. Instead, pay good attention to the quality of your protein source.

Tip: If you are unsure which protein shake is healthy, try our Primal Collagen Cacao. It consists of 100% natural ingredients.

4. Fruits and berries

Although fruits contain vitamins and minerals, they often also contain large amounts of fructose. You can measure the effect on your ketosis. Therefore, we focus in this section, especially on berries.

Allowed:

Blueberries, strawberries, blackberries, raspberries, elderberries, currants, avocado, papaya

Recommendation: Focus on low-sugar fruits such as berries. Treat her like some sweets. For example, you can make a delicious berry sorbet with frozen blueberries for dessert.

5. Drinks

Water, water with lemon juice, herbal tea, coffee, high-quality green tea, homemade lemonade, homemade ice tea, coconut milk, and almond milk (unsweetened)

Recommendation: It is essential to drink enough water. Try to take at least 2-3 liters of fluid daily.

6. Nuts and seeds

Macadamia, almond, coconut, pecans, walnuts, and cashews

Recommendation: Since nuts are rich in trace elements, but also contain anti-nutrients such as phytic acid, you should limit the consumption to a handful per day.

7. Spices and herbs

Cider vinegar, Ceylon cinnamon, coriander, cocoa powder, coconut amino (if tolerated), ginger, mustard, oregano, parsley, rosemary, sea salt, thyme, turmeric, vanilla pod

Recommendation: No matter which nutritional form you choose. Be it the low carb diet or a ketogenic diet, spices and herbs have their place. Pay attention to the highest possible quality and refrain from artificial additives.

8. Ketogenic alternatives

Keto Mayonnaise, Keto Biscuits, 85% Chocolate, Keto Cocoa, Keto Energy Balls, Keto Gummy Bears,

Recommendation: It is always practical to have delicious and ketogenic alternatives to the small sins of the diet at home. For example, in our office, we always have ketogenic mayonnaise and ketogenic biscuits.

FOODS TO AVOID

Of course, you should be careful to keep your consumption of carbohydrates low in a ketogenic diet. But by now, you have also learned that we are not only concerned with the macronutrients, but also the quality of the food to eat and the effect on your health.

Here you can find out which foods are not part of a healthy ketogenic diet.

1. Sugar in all forms

Sugar (sucrose), corn syrup (GFS, HFCS), agave syrup, molasses, brown sugar, granulated sugar, cane sugar, caramel, coconut sugar, palm sugar, sugarcane juice, fruit juice, fruit juice concentrate, sugar beet syrup, glucose, invert sugar, molasses

Ketogenic alternative: xylitol, erythritol, stevia, ribose, primal sweet

2. Artificial additives / food

Artificial flavors, artificial colors, artificial sugar substitutes, trans fat, bouillon

Ketogenic alternative: real ingredients that provide real flavors!

3. Cereal products

Cereal products contain large amounts of fast carbohydrates and will immediately kick you out of ketosis. Therefore, you should avoid them. This includes:

Bread, pasta, cake, biscuits, pizza, cornmeal

Tip: You do not have to do without tasty pasta entirely if you know the right alternatives. For example, there is super delicious gluten-free bread or ketogenic spaghetti.

Alternatives: coconut flour, almond flour

Chapter 10: Basic shopping list

Onion

Olive oil

Mushrooms or ten ounces chopped

One block firm organic tofu in water drained and then pressed for a few minutes

Fresh spinach

One red pepper chopped

Garlic powder

A little veggie broth

Pepper to taste

One-half tsp. of turmeric

Pinch paprika optional

Garlic cloves minced - three

Italian seasoning

The juice of one lemon

One-fourth cup of unsalted butter - melted

Two medium zucchini - cut these diagonally into one half inch slices

Chopped fresh parsley leaves

Fresh ground pepper

kosher salt

Keto sweetener

Some butter or any nut butter or even coconut oil

Vanilla extract

Pinch of salt

Almond flour

Coconut flour

Heavy whipping cream or coconut cream

Butter

MCT oil

Coffee

Mushroom coffee

Almond flour

Baking powder

Mozzarella, grated

Cream cheese

Eggs

Chapter 11: Breakfast Recipes

Bulletproof Coffee

Ingredients:

1 tsp butter

1 tsp MCT oil

250 ml of coffee (or mushroom coffee), this is gentler on the stomach and additionally promotes fat burning in the long term)

Mushroom coffee:

Ingredients:

145g almond flour

1 tbsp baking powder

283g mozzarella, grated

56g cream cheese

2 (L) eggs

Optional for topping - sesame seeds

Directions

Preheat the oven to 200 ° C and layout the baking tray with baking paper.

Mix almond flour and baking powder and set aside.

Put mozzarella and cream cheese in a large bowl and microwave for 2 minutes. Stir briefly after one minute and stir again after 2 minutes.

If you do not have a microwave, then heat the cheese on a double griddle on the stove over low heat, constantly stirring, until completely melted.

Put the flour mixture and the eggs in the melted cheese.

Tip: Here, you have to be fast; the cheese must be still hot.

Knead everything well with your hands until a dough forms.

The dough will be very sticky, but do not let it irritate you - knead and squeeze the dough with your fingers for a few minutes.

If the dough becomes hard before it is thoroughly mixed, you can microwave it for 15-20 seconds and heat it to soften it. In this case, wash your hands again before starting to knead the dough again.

Divide the dough into 6 pieces and form a long "sausage" out of each piece of dough. Squeeze the ends together to form the bagel shape.

Put the bagel dough pieces on the baking sheet. If you still want to use sesame as a topping, sprinkle it over the bagels and gently squeeze them into the dough.

Bake the bagels for 10-14 minutes.

Ketogenic protein bars

Ingredients:

125 ml Nut from Brazil Nuts (2 Handfuls) & Macadamia Nuts (1 Large Handful) & Pecans (1 Handful)

80 ml grated coconut flakes (here are the cheap ones from the baking department)

80 g hemp protein powder (excellent low in the cow and good fat content)

1 tbsp almond flour (de-oiled)

0.5 packet of baking powder

1 egg

If too friable, then add a dash of unsweetened almond milk, so you can just put the dough in the protein bar molds.

Optional at the end bittersweet chocolate 70 - 85% chocolate

Directions

Process all nuts in the blender to make mus

Then destroy all the dry ingredients in a bowl.

Add the egg, and then mix the sweetener and nutmeg with the other ingredients.

Either fill everything in a muffin case as in the video or distribute it flat on a baking sheet and then cut into bars

Approximately Cook for 20-30 minutes at 180 degrees (depends on how you shaped them, the flatter the shorter the baking time)

Just before the end of the chocolate over it and lightly melt.

pizza waffles

Ingredients:

4 eggs (L)

4 tablespoons of grated Parmesan

1 tbsp butter

3 tablespoons almond flour

85g cheddar cheese

1 teaspoon Baking powder

1 tablespoon of psyllium powder

salt and pepper

Optional:

1 tsp Italian spice, e.g., oregano

Tomato sauce, without sugar

14 salami slices (optional)

Directions

All ingredients except the tomato sauce and cheese in a bowl and mix well with a hand mixer.

Put the dough on your waffle iron as usual.

Spread the finished waffle with the tomato sauce (about ¼ cup per waffle) and the cheese. Optionally you can add a few salami slices to the waffle pizza.

Now bake the waffle pizza for 3-5 minutes in the oven at about 150 degrees until the cheese has melted.

Low-carb coconut juice

Ingredients:

2 tbsp coconut flour

optional: 2 tbsp linseed

180 ml of water or milk

pinch of salt

1 large egg, beaten

2 tsp butter

1 tbsp coconut milk

1/2 tbsp Steviala Crystal

Directions

Take a small saucepan and add the coconut flour, linseed, salt, and the water. Heat the contents of the pan, stirring over low heat until it starts to thicken.

Take away the pan from the heat and add half of the beaten egg. Stir well and then add the other half. Then place the pan on the heat and heat, stirring, until it starts to take on the porridge structure.

Release the pan from the heat and add the butter, coconut milk, and Stevia Crystal while stirring. Pour the contents into a small bowl and serve with fresh fruit!

Broccoli and cheese muffins

Ingredients:

600 g broccoli florets

7 eggs, only the protein

4 large whole eggs

30 g of grated cheddar cheese

40 g of grated cheese of your choice

1 tbsp of olive oil

salt and pepper to taste

Directions

Preheat the oven to 180 degrees. Pour a small amount of water in a pan and steam in the broccoli florets for about 6-7 minutes. Now take a bowl and break the broccoli florets into smaller pieces after cooking. Add the olive oil and salt and pepper to taste and mix this well with the broccoli florets.

Grease a muffin mold with 9 molds with butter. Divide the broccoli florets evenly over the 9 molds. Grab another bowl and beat in the eggs, egg whites, grated cheese, and mix well.

Now also divide the egg mixture evenly over the 9 molds and finally sprinkle the grated cheddar cheese over the molds. Bake the broccoli and cheese muffins for about 20 minutes in the preheated oven.

Tofu Scramble with Sweet Potatoes

Ingredients:

For sweet potatoes:

- ¾ pound sweet potatoes, scrubbed, chopped into ½ inch cubes

- Salt to taste

- Pepper to taste

- ½ tablespoon olive oil

- 1 teaspoon chili powder

For tofu scramble:

- 1 tablespoon olive oil

- ½ package (from a 14 ounces package) extra-firm tofu, drained, crumbled

- 1 small onion, chopped

- 1 cup chopped asparagus

- ½ teaspoon garlic powder

- 1 bell pepper, deseed if desired, finely chopped

- Salt to taste

- Pepper to taste

- ½ teaspoon ground cumin

- ½ teaspoon turmeric powder

Directions:

Add sweet potatoes into a bowl. Sprinkle salt, pepper and chili powder and toss well. Drizzle oil and toss well.

Transfer onto a lined baking sheet. Spread it evenly.

Bake in a preheated oven at 425° F for 30 minutes or until cooked through. Stir once halfway through baking.

Place a skillet over medium-high heat. Add oil. When the oil is heated, add onion, asparagus and bell pepper. Sauté for 6-7 minutes or until tender.

Stir in the tofu, spices, and salt. Heat thoroughly.

Take 3 – 4 meal prep containers and divide the scramble among them.

Also divide the sweet potatoes among the containers.

Refrigerate until use. It can last for 4 days.

Carrot Cake Quinoa Breakfast Bars

Ingredients:

For wet ingredients:

- 2 flax eggs (2 tablespoons of ground flaxseed mixed with 6 tablespoons water)

- 1 cup mashed banana

- 2 cups cooked or canned chickpeas

- 1 cup unsweetened applesauce

For dry ingredients:

- 1 ½ cups quinoa flour

- 2 teaspoons ground cinnamon

- 1 teaspoon ground vanilla bean or 2 teaspoons pure vanilla extract

- 1/8 teaspoon salt

- 1 cup coconut sugar

- 1 teaspoon ground nutmeg

- 1 teaspoon baking soda

For add-ins:

- ½ cup hemp hearts

- ½ cup chopped walnuts

- 1 cup grated carrots

Optional toppings:

- Chopped walnuts

Directions:

Take a large baking dish (13 x 9 inches) and grease with some cooking spray. Place a sheet of parchment paper in it.

Once you mix the water and ground flaxseed, set aside for 15 minutes.

Add the rest of the wet ingredients into a blender and blend until smooth.

Add all the dry ingredients into a mixing bowl and stir.

Add the wet ingredients and flax eggs into the bowl of dry ingredients and mix until well incorporated.

Add hemp hearts, walnuts and carrots and fold gently.

Pour the batter into the baking dish.

Bake in a preheated oven at 350° F for 23 – 27 minutes. The cake is ready when a toothpick inserted in the center does not have any particles stuck on it when removed from the cake.

Remove the baking dish from the oven. Take out the cake from the dish after 15 – 20 minutes and place on a wire rack.

Let it cool to room temperature.

Cut into 30 – 32 equal pieces. Transfer into an airtight container. It can last for 2 – 3 days at room temperature or for 5 – 6 days in the refrigerator.

Oven Baked Beans

Ingredients:

- ½ tablespoon olive oil

- 1 red onion, chopped

- 1 small red chili, deseeded, finely chopped

- ½ teaspoon smoked paprika

- ¼ teaspoon ground cumin

- ½ teaspoon chili flakes

- 2 – 3 sprigs fresh thyme

- 12 ounces tomato passata

- 1 tablespoon balsamic vinegar

- ¼ teaspoon Tabasco sauce (optional)

- 1 can (15 ounces) white beans like pinto beans or borlotti beans, drained, rinsed

- ½ teaspoon molasses

- 2 cloves garlic, peeled, minced

- Salt to taste

- Pepper to taste

Directions:

Add onion, chili, and garlic into a baking dish. Drizzle oil over it. Add all the spices and toss well.

Cover the baking dish with aluminum foil.

Bake in a preheated oven at 340° F for 20 minutes.

Remove the dish from the oven and uncover.

Add rest of the ingredients and mix well. If you find the mixture very dry, add a little water and mix well.

Bake for 30 – 40 minutes. Do not cover the dish while baking.

Remove from the oven and cool completely.

Transfer into an airtight container and refrigerate until use. It can last for 5 days. If you want to freeze it, place in freezer bags and freeze until use. It can last for 3 months.

To serve: Thaw if frozen. Heat thoroughly in an oven or microwave.

Serve with toasted bread if desired.

Zucchini Muffins

Serves: 9

Ingredients:

For wet ingredients:

- ¼ cup lightly packed dark brown sugar

- ¾ cup grated zucchini

- ¼ cup granulated organic sugar

- 3 tablespoons unsweetened applesauce

- 2 tablespoons canola oil

- 6 tablespoons almond milk

For dry ingredients:

- ¼ cup almond meal

- ¾ cup + 2 tablespoons white spelt flour

- ½ teaspoon baking powder

- ½ teaspoon baking soda

- ½ teaspoon ground cinnamon

- ¼ teaspoon salt

- 1/8 teaspoon ground nutmeg

Directions:

Add all the wet ingredients into a mixing bowl and whisk well. Se
aside for 5 minutes.

Add all the dry ingredients into another bowl and stir.

Add the mixture of dry ingredients into the bowl of wet ingredient:
and mix until well combined. Do not over mix.

Take 9 muffin cups and grease with olive oil. Place disposable muffir
liners in it. Divide the batter into the prepared muffin cups.

Bake in a preheated oven at 350° F for 20 – 25 minutes or a toothpick
when inserted in the center of the muffin comes out clean. Remove the
muffins from the mold and place on a wire rack. Cool completely.

Store in an airtight container at room temperature for up to 2 days.
You can refrigerate the muffins. It can last for 4-5 days.

To freeze: Wrap individual muffins in plastic wrap. Place the muffins
in freezer-safe bags. Freeze until use. It can last for 1 month in the
freezer.

To serve: Thaw the muffins completely and warm for a few seconds in
the microwave before serving.

Potato and Tofu Tacos

Ingredients:

- 1 tablespoon vegetable oil

- ½ large bell pepper, diced

- 3 strips vegan bacon

- ½ tablespoon nutritional yeast

- Himalayan pink salt to taste

- 6 flour tortillas

- 1 medium onion, diced

- 1 cup frozen, diced potatoes

- 1 block firm tofu, drained, pressed of excess moisture, crumbled

- ½ teaspoon garlic powder

- Pepper to taste

- Salt to taste

Directions:

Place a large skillet over medium heat. Add ½ tablespoon of oil. When the oil is heated, add onion and bell pepper and sauté until onion turns translucent.

Stir in the potatoes and mix well.

Lower the heat to low heat and cover with a lid. Cook until potatoes are well cooked. Stir every 5 minutes. Add salt and pepper to taste. Transfer into a bowl and let it cool.

Add ½ tablespoon oil into the skillet. When the oil is heated, add tofu and cook until nearly dry.

Stir in the vegan bacon. Cook until tofu is light brown. Add nutritional yeast and garlic powder.

Remove from heat. Add Himalayan pink salt and pepper and mix well.

Spread the tortillas on your countertop. Divide the potatoes and tofu among the tortillas. Roll and wrap in aluminum foil.

Place the wrapped tacos in freezer-safe bags. Freeze until use. It can last for 15 days.

To serve: Remove from the oven and discard the foil. Wrap the taco in paper towel and place in a microwave. Cook on high for a minute or until heated through.

Serve with salsa or any other dip of your choice.

Vegan Strata

Ingredients:

- ½ tablespoon German mustard

- ¼ cup vegetable broth or water

- ½ cup finely chopped celery

- ½ cup finely chopped onion

- 2 ounces mushrooms, thinly sliced

- 7 ounces vegan beef crumbles

- 1 cup vegan mozzarella cheese shreds

- 1 cup chopped spinach

- 2 ½ cups diced sourdough bread

For vegan egg batter:

- ¾ cup chickpea flour

- 1 tablespoon flaxseed meal

- ½ teaspoon salt

- Pepper to taste

- A large pinch nutmeg

- 1 ½ cups unsweetened almond milk

- 1 tablespoon nutritional yeast

- ½ teaspoon turmeric powder

- ¼ teaspoon Himalayan pink salt or to taste

Serving day ingredients:

- 2 tablespoons chopped parsley

- 1 green onion, thinly sliced

Directions:

Spray a 6-inch freezer safe, baking dish with cooking spray.

Place a nonstick skillet over medium flame. Add broth. When the broth is heated, add mushrooms, celery and onion and cook until onions are pink.

Add vegan sausage and stir. Break it simultaneously as it cooks. Add more broth if the mixture is stuck to the bottom of the pan. Turn off the heat.

Add mustard and spinach and mix well.

To make vegan egg batter: Add all the ingredients for vegan egg batter into a bowl and whisk well.

Spread the sausage mixture on the bottom of the prepared baking dish.

Scatter bread pieces and cheese. Pour egg batter and mix the sausage mixture, bread and cheese until well coated.

Cover the dish with cling wrap. Chill overnight.

Bake in a preheated oven at 350° F for about 45 – 50 minutes or until set.

Let it cool to room temperature.

Sprinkle green onion and parsley on top and serve.

Vegan Sausage Breakfast Lasagna

Ingredients:

- 4.5 ounces no-boil lasagna noodles

- 3 scallions, thinly sliced

- 4 ounces vegan mozzarella cheese shreds

For béchamel sauce:

- ¼ cup unbleached all-purpose flour

- 1 medium leek, green and white parts only

- 8 ounces frozen chopped spinach

- ½ teaspoon dried oregano

- ½ teaspoon dried sage

- 2 cloves garlic, minced

- 2 cups cashew milk or any other vegan milk of your choice

- Salt to taste

- Pepper to taste

- ½ tablespoon extra-virgin olive oil

- ¼ teaspoon ground nutmeg

- 7 ounces vegan Italian sausages, chopped

Directions:

To make béchamel sauce: Place a skillet over medium heat. Add oil. When the oil is heated, add leeks and garlic and sauté for a minute and cook until tender.

Stir in the sausages, salt, pepper, oregano, sage, and nutmeg.

Stir in the flour and sauté for a couple of minutes.

Pour cashew milk, stirring constantly. Continue stirring until thick. When the sauce begins to boil, turn off the heat.

To assemble: Take a baking dish of about 8 inches. Spoon some of the béchamel sauce on the bottom of the baking dish. Spread a layer of noodles (about 2-3) over the sauce layer.

Layer with half the spinach. Spread a little béchamel sauce over the spinach followed by 1/3 the cheese and 1/3 the scallions.

Place remaining noodles over the scallions.

Follow step 6 again.

Spread the remaining sauce on top. Scatter remaining cheese and scallions.

Cover the dish with plastic wrap.

Refrigerate until use. It can last for 2-3 days.

Remove the baking dish from the refrigerator and discard plastic wrap. Cover the dish with foil.

Bake in a preheated oven at 350° F for about 30 minutes. Uncover and bake until the top is golden brown.

Remove from the oven and let it rest for 5-7 minutes.

Serve hot, warm or cold.

Quinoa Breakfast Tacos

Serves: 8

Ingredients:

For quinoa:

- 3 cups cooked quinoa

- 2 tablespoons fresh lime juice

- ½ cup chopped cilantro

- Salt to taste

- Freshly ground pepper to taste

For butternut squash:

- 4 tablespoons coconut oil

- 1 bunch Swiss chard or kale, discard hard stems and ribs, finely chopped

- 8 cups cubed butternut squash

- Salt to taste

- Freshly ground pepper to taste

- 1 teaspoon chili powder

Serving day ingredients:

- 16 tortillas

- 8 scallions, thinly sliced

- 2 large ripe avocados, pitted, peeled, thinly sliced

- Salt to taste

- Freshly ground pepper to taste

- 2 cups shredded red cabbage

Directions:

To make quinoa: Add all the ingredients for quinoa into an airtight container and mix well. Close the lid and refrigerate until use.

To make filling: Place a large skillet over medium heat. Add oil. When the oil is heated, add squash and cook for about 8 minutes.

Add rest of the ingredients for the filling and cook until kale wilts. Remove from heat and cool completely. Transfer into an airtight container and refrigerate until use. The filling and quinoa can store for 4 days.

To serve: Remove the quinoa and filling from the refrigerator and warm it in the microwave. Heat the tortillas following the directions on the package.

Place the tortillas on individual serving plates. Divide the quinoa, butternut squash filling, scallions, avocados and cabbage among the tortillas. Season with salt and pepper and serve.

Blueberry Baked Oatmeal

Ingredients:

- 1/3 cup chopped pecans

- 1 teaspoon ground cinnamon

- 1/8 teaspoon ground nutmeg

- 3 tablespoons maple syrup

- 1 ½ tablespoons coconut oil, melted

- 6 ounces blueberries, fresh or frozen, divided

- 1 cup old fashioned oats

- ½ teaspoon baking powder

- ¾ cup + 2 tablespoons nondairy milk of your choice, at room temperature

- 1 teaspoon vanilla extract

- 1 teaspoon raw sugar (optional)

Optional toppings: Use any

- Vegan vanilla yogurt

- Blueberries

- 1 flax egg

- Vegan whipped cream

- Maple syrup

- Any other toppings of your choice

Directions:

After mixing the flaxseeds with water, set aside for 15 minutes.

Take a square baking dish of about 6 x 6 and grease with cooking spray. Set aside.

Spread pecans on a rimmed baking sheet.

Bake in a preheated oven at 375° F for 4 – 5 minutes or until toasted and aromatic.

Transfer into a mixing bowl. Also add in the oats, cinnamon, salt, baking powder and nutmeg. Stir until well incorporated.

Add milk, flax egg, maple syrup, vanilla, and coconut oil into a bowl and whisk well.

Set aside ¼ cup of blueberries and place the rest of the berries in the prepared baking dish. Spread it evenly.

Spread the oat mixture over the berries. Spoon the milk mixture over the oat layer. Lightly tap the dish on your countertop.

Press lightly on the oats so that it is soaked in milk.

Sprinkle the berries (that were set aside) on top. Scatter sugar on top.

Bake in a preheated oven at 375° F for 30 minutes or until golden brown on top.

Take out the dish from the oven and let it cool to room temperature.

Cover the dish with foil and refrigerate until use. It can last for 4 – 5 days.

To serve: Cut into portions and place in a microwave-safe bowl. Heat thoroughly and serve.

Strawberry Banana Spinach Smoothie

Ingredients:

For smoothie:

- 1 cup frozen, sliced bananas

- 2 cups fresh spinach

- 1 cup frozen whole strawberries

- 2 teaspoons chia seeds

Serving day ingredients (per smoothie bag):

- Unsweetened almond milk, as required

- 1 scoop vegan vanilla protein powder

Directions:

Divide all the ingredients for the smoothie into 2 Ziploc bags. Squeeze the bag to remove any air. Seal the bag. Label the bag with the date and name of the smoothie. Freeze until use. It can last for 3 months.

Serving day: Remove a bag from the freezer and thaw slightly if desired. Add all the contents of the bag into a high-speed blender.

Add milk and protein powder. Blend until smooth.

Pour into a glass and serve.

Breakfast Cookies

Ingredients:

For wet ingredients:

- 1 medium overripe bananas, mashed

- 1 tablespoon maple syrup

- 1 flax egg (1 tablespoon ground flax seeds mixed with tablespoons water)

- ¼ cup creamy, unsalted, peanut butter

- 1 tablespoon melted coconut oil

- ½ teaspoon pure vanilla extract

For dry ingredients:

- 1 cup gluten-free rolled oats

- ¼ teaspoon baking soda

- ¼ teaspoon baking powder

Add-ins:

- ¼ cup finely chopped walnuts

- ¼ cup raisins

Optional toppings:

- 1 tablespoon chopped walnuts

- 1 tablespoons raisins

Directions:

Once you mix the water and ground flaxseed, set aside for 15 minutes

Add all the wet ingredients into a bowl and stir until well incorporated

Mix together all the dry ingredients in another bowl. Add the dry ingredients into the bowl of wet ingredients. Mix well into a dough.

Divide the dough into 12 – 15 equal portions. Sprinkle optional toppings if using.

Bake in a preheated oven at 350° F for 12-15 minutes or until light golden brown.

Remove from the oven and let the cookies cool for 7 – 8 minutes on the baking sheet. Loosen the cookies with a metal spatula.

Cool completely. Transfer into an airtight container. It can be stored at room temperature for 4 to 5 days. For longer, store the container in the refrigerator. It can last for 10 – 12 days. For even longer, transfer into freezer-safe bags. Label the bags and freeze for up to 2 months.

Chia pudding with coconut and strawberries

Ingredients:

250 ml unsweetened almond milk or coconut milk

3 tbsp chia seeds (25 g)

2 tbsp ground coconut

1 tsp vanilla aroma

1 handful of strawberries, cut into pieces

Stevia or erythritol to taste

Directions

In a large bowl, combine the almond milk, ground coconut, chia seed, sweetener and the vanilla aroma with a whisk. Divide the mixture over

2 dishes and let it stand for 10 minutes. Stir everything together occasionally during the 10 minutes. Place the 2 dishes in the fridge all night or for at least 2 hours and place the strawberries on the pudding before serving.

Low carbohydrate French toast

Ingredients:

37 g coconut flour

25 g Steviala Crystal

6 medium eggs

100 ml of almond milk

2 tsp baking powder

1 tsp cinnamon

1 tsp vanilla aroma

35 g butter

40 ml of cream

pinch of salt

Directions

In a big bowl, mix the coconut flour, Steviala crystal, baking powder, cinnamon, and a pinch of salt. Take another bowl and mix in 4 eggs, 50 ml almond milk, and the vanilla flavor. Then add the flour mix to the egg mix and beat until it smoothens.

Then add the melted butter to the batter and keep stirring. Then grease 4 small dishes or ramekins with a little butter or olive oil. Divide the batter between the four dishes and then put them in the microwave (800 watts) for 5 minutes.

Meanwhile, mix the remaining eggs, almond milk, and cream in another bowl. Add any cinnamon to taste and beat until whole. Remove the rolls from the microwave after 5 minutes and let them cool for at least 1.5 minutes.

Cut the buns in half and dip each half well in the creamy batter. Then heat a tbsp of butter and bake the French toast golden brown. Serve the French toast with fresh fruit and possibly some Steviala Frost!

Ketogenic muffins as spinach quiche

Ingredients:

Olive oil - for the champions

1 pack of fresh spinach (we prefer to use the baby spinach, about 285g)

4 medium-sized eggs

1 cup of grated cheese (we use mozzarella here)

1 pack of brown champions (minced)

1-2 tablespoons whipped cream

Salt and pepper to taste

Strong - Variation:

Directions

Preheat the oven to 180 ° C.

Heat a little oil in a large pan and fry the mushrooms until soft (about 5-6 minutes). Set the champions aside.

Put the spinach in a slightly deeper pan or take the pan that you have already used for the mushrooms.

Add ¼ cup of water to the spinach. Now boil for 3-4 minutes on medium. Make sure the spinach does not wither.

Afterward, thoroughly drain the excess water from the spinach.

Whisk the eggs in a large mixing bowl with a whisk.

Add the mushrooms, spinach, cheese, and cream to the eggs. Mix everything well.

Taste the mixture with salt and pepper.

Now spread everything on 12 muffin cases and put the muffins in the preheated oven for 20-25 minutes. It's best to test the toothpick after 20 minutes.

Sprinkle some more cheese on top.

Cloud Bread

Ingredients:

Ketogenic cloud bread

3 eggs

3 tablespoons cream cheese

¼ Tl baking powder

for cloud french toast

6-8 slices of cloud bread

2 eggs

50g milk or cream

50g erythritol (sugar replacement)

1 teaspoon cinnamon

½ tsp vanilla extract

salt

2 teaspoons butter

Topping variants: maple syrup, fresh raspberries

Directions

Short info about the delicious cloud bread:

In a low carb / ketogenic diet, normal bread should be removed from the diet - it contains too many carbohydrates. We have found the perfect solution, as you do not have to give up your bread. The "cloud bread" is keto-friendly and an ideal alternative to regular bread. Here is completely dispensed with flour.

Bread recipe: cloud bread

Separate the egg white from the egg yolk.

Mix the cream cheese with the egg yolk in a bowl.

In another bowl, the baking powder is stirred under the egg white and then beaten stiff.

Gently lift the egg yolks cream cheese mass under the egg whites and stir everything into homogenous dough.

Layout your baking tray with baking paper. Now make small patties or a larger bread from the dough.

Put the bread or patties in the oven for about 15 minutes at 150 degrees

French Cloud Toast

Mix eggs, milk or cream, sugar, cinnamon, vanilla extract, and a pinch of salt in a shallow bowl (or deep dish).

Place 1 or 2 pieces of cloud bread in the ready-mixed liquid to soak. Turn the slices of bread in about a minute.

Heat the butter at medium speed until it has melted. Now put the cloud bread slices in the pan and fry them on each side until they are slightly golden brown.

Serve the cloud french toast with maple syrup and raspberries.

Frittata Pizza

Ingredients:

12 eggs (L)

250g spinach (TK)

2 medium-hot peppers

140g mozzarella

1 teaspoon finely chopped garlic (if you do not want to eat garlic in the morning, you can omit it)

125g ricotta

55g Parmesan

4 tablespoons olive oil

¼ tsp nutmeg

Salt & pepper to taste

Directions

First, prepare the spinach according to the package instructions. Try to make sure that you drain as much water as possible later. Set the spinach aside.

Preheat your oven to 190 ° C.

Mix eggs, olive oil, and the spices together.

Add the ricotta, Parmesan cheese, and spinach (should not be hot).

Pour the mixture into a cast-iron skillet and sprinkle with the mozzarella and hot peppers above.

Now bake the pizza frittata for 30 minutes.

If you use a glass baking dish, the baking time will be extended by about 10-15 minutes.

apple cinnamon bars

Apple cinnamon protein bar

Ingredients:

4 eggs

1 cup of ground pecans

52g coconut oil

¼ cup of freeze-dried apples

2 teaspoons cinnamon

1 tsp vanilla extract

10 drops of liquid Stevia

Directions

First, preheat your oven to 180 ° C.

If you do not have ground pecans, then put the nuts in your blender and grind them finely.

Place eggs, coconut oil, vanilla, stevia, and cinnamon in a mixing bowl. Mix everything thoroughly.

Add nuts and the dried apples (very small pieces) and mix everything together.

Pour the batter into a pan and bake for 25 minutes. It's best to do the wood stick test!

Chapter 12: Lunch RecipesKeto Lasagna

Ingredients:

1 tbsp butter or coconut oil

1 egg

200 g of chorizo or Italian salami

400 g ricotta

2 tablespoons coconut flour

1 ½ teaspoon sea salt

½ tsp pepper

2 garlic cloves, pressed

1 ½ cups mozzarella, grated

⅓ cup of Parmesan, grated

4 zucchini, cut into fine strips

500 g Italian tomato sauce

1 teaspoon Italian herbs

¼ cup of basil

Directions

Heat butter or coconut oil in a pan and fry the sausage in it. Then remove from the pan and let cool.

Preheat oven to 200 degrees and grease a baking pan with a little butter or coconut oil.

Put the ricotta, mozzarella, 2 tablespoons of Parmesan cheese, 1 egg, coconut flour, salt, garlic and pepper in a bowl and mix well.

Add the Italian herbs and marina sauce and stir well.

Put a layer of zucchini in the baking pan.

Add a layer of cheese mixture and season with Italian herbs. Then add a layer of marinara and repeat 3-4 times.

Bake the lasagne in the oven for about 30-40 minutes.

Remove from the oven and garnish with fresh basil if necessary.

Keto California Rolls

Ingredients:

1 cucumber

100 g salmon, chopped

350 g cauliflower, finely chopped (about rice grain size)

60 g cream cheese

1 avocado, thinly sliced

1 teaspoon sesame oil

1 teaspoon mayonnaise

sea-salt

Roasted sesame seeds

Directions

Cut the cucumber lengthwise into very fine slices. Then place slices on some kitchen paper and let it dry a bit.

Fry the chopped cauliflower in a pan until tender. Stir in cream cheese and sesame oil and mix well.

Salmon in a bowl and mix with the mayonnaise.

Take some cling film and place the cucumber slices on the foil.

Put "Blumkohlreis" and the rest of the stuffing on the cucumber slices.

Firmly roll the cucumber slices together using the cling film and make 4 sushi rolls.

Put the sushi rolls in the fridge for one hour.

Remove sushi rolls from the refrigerator and cut them into pieces. Then serve sushi with wasabi and soy sauce and garnish with a little roasted sesame.

Egg wrap with salmon and spinach

Ingredients:

3 medium eggs

dash of almond milk

100 gr baby spinach

2 tbsp olive oil

salt and pepper to taste

25 g cream cheese

20 g arugula

50 gr smoked salmon

4 cherry tomatoes

1/4 tsp salt

optional: a handful of pine nuts

Directions

Cut the baby spinach into small pieces on a large board. Heat a little tablespoon of olive oil in a medium-sized frying pan and fry the baby spinach approximately. 2 minutes. Mix the eggs, almond milk, and salt in a large bowl with a whisk. After frying the spinach, drain the excess from the pan and add the spinach to the bowl and mix well with the eggs.

In the same frying pan, fry the spinach omelet over low heat for 5-10 minutes until cooked. If possible, carefully turn the omelet halfway through baking with a spatula.

Allow the omelet to cool for a minimum of 30 minutes and then cut the cherry tomatoes into small slices. When the omelet has cooled, spread the cream cheese over the omelet and coated with the arugula, smoked salmon, cherry tomatoes, and pine nuts. Roll the omelet tightly, cut in half and enjoy!

Thai Beef Salad/Thai steal salad

Ingredients:

Marinade

2 tsp grated ginger

2 cloves of garlic

1/2 teaspoon chopped lemongrass (Go-Tan)

1/2 shallot, very finely sliced

2 tbsp fish sauce

optional: 1 tsp honey

Salad

300 gr steak

200 g romaine lettuce

1 shallot

2 stalks of spring onion

hand fresh mint

1 red or green bell pepper

1 cucumber

3 tbsp peanuts or cashews

30 gr butter for baking or roasting

Dressing

2 tbsp soy sauce

1 tbsp fish sauce

2 tbsp lime juice

1 tsp grated ginger

optional: 1 tsp honey

Directions

To make the marinade, add the ginger, garlic, lemongrass, shallot, and fish sauce to a blender and blend it on until everything is well mixed. Then take a fresh food container and put the steak in here. Pour the marinade over the beef and close the container. Put the container in the fridge and let the marinade withdraw for at least an hour.

Then, on a wide cutting board, cut the romaine lettuce, spring onion, cucumber, bell pepper, mint, shallot, and peanuts into small pieces, and divide this into two bowls.

Remove the marinated steak from the refrigerator and let it rest for 15 minutes at room temperature. Then subject the butter to heat in a frying pan and add the steak to the pan when the foam disappears. Bake the steak 2-3 minutes per side or, if desired, rare, medium or well done.

Meanwhile, make the dressing by mixing the soy sauce, fish sauce, lime juice, and ginger in a small bowl. Then cut the fried steak into strips and divide this together with the dressing between the two bowls. Enjoy your meal!

Miso Glazed Sweet Potato Bowls

Ingredients:

- 1 medium sweet potato, peeled, cut into 2-inch cubes (about 2 cups)

- ½ teaspoon turmeric powder

- 1 tablespoon tamari

- 1 tablespoon pure maple syrup

- ½ onion, finely chopped

- ½ teaspoon garlic powder

- 4 ounces mushrooms, finely chopped

- ¾ cup uncooked farro

- 1 ½ tablespoons white miso

- ½ tablespoon rice wine vinegar

- ½ tablespoon extra-virgin olive oil

- 1 large bunch kale, discard hard stems and ribs

- Salt to taste

- Pepper to taste

- Water, as required

Serving day ingredients:

- Avocado slices

- Tahini sauce

Directions:

Spread the sweet potatoes on a lined baking sheet.

Bake in a preheated oven at 425° F for about 20 minutes. Stir once halfway through baking.

Place a saucepan with 1-½ cups of water over medium heat. Bring to a boil.

Add farro and cook until tender and dry. Add more water if it is not cooked. Stir in the turmeric. Turn off the heat and fluff with a fork. Let it cool completely.

Place a pot over medium heat. Add oil. When the oil is heated, add onion and sauté until translucent.

Stir in the mushrooms, salt, garlic powder and pepper and cook until slightly brown.

Add kale and mix well. Cook until it wilts.

Add miso, vinegar, 2 – 3 tablespoons water, tamari and maple syrup into a bowl and whisk well.

Add the roasted sweet potatoes into the bowl of sauce mixture. Stir until well coated.

Divide into 2 meal prep containers. Divide the farro and mushroom – kale mixture among the containers and refrigerate until use. It can last for 3 – 4 days.

To serve: Serve warm or at room temperature with avocado and tahini sauce on top.

Low carbohydrate cauliflower couscous

Ingredients:

600 g cauliflower florets

75 g sundried tomatoes

1 - 2 cloves of garlic, crushed

1 tbsp olive oil

150 g leek, finely chopped

salt and pepper to taste

pinch of paprika powder

pinch of finely ground cumin

1 tbsp lemon juice

50 g walnuts, chopped into pieces

optional: feta cheese to taste

Directions

Take a bowl of water and soak the sun-dried tomatoes in it. Then put the cauliflower florets in a food processor and grind granular, just like real couscous. Add lemon juice to the cauliflower and season with pepper, salt, cumin, and paprika powder.

Take a medium-sized frying pan and heat a tablespoon of olive oil in it. Add the finely crushed garlic cloves and the leek pieces and cook for a few minutes over medium heat.

In the meantime, take the container with sun-dried tomatoes and drain the water. Cut the sun-dried tomatoes into small pieces and add to the frying pan.

Add the cauliflower couscous and the walnuts to the pan and cook until done. Make sure you do not bake it for too long because then it will become a porridge. Divide over four plates and enjoy!

Stuffed courgettes with tuna

Ingredients:

2 medium-sized courgettes

1 small onion

1/2 red pepper

150 g canned tuna in oil

1 clove of garlic, crushed

70 g grated Parmesan cheese

Directions

Preheat the oven to 180 degrees. Cut the two zucchini into half and scoop them out with a spoon. You don't need the flesh, and you can use it for a different recipe.

Then cut the bell pepper, onion, and garlic into small pieces on a board. Take the can of tuna and drain a large part of the oil. Then take a medium-sized bowl and add the tuna. Add the finely chopped vegetables and mix everything well together.

Divide the tuna mixture over the four hollowed-out zucchini pieces and garnish with parmesan cheese, pepper, and salt. Then put the zucchini pieces in the oven for 15 minutes. Enjoy your meal!

Tofu Burrito Bowl

Ingredients:

- ½ package (from a 14 ounces package) extra-firm tofu, drained, pressed of excess moisture, chopped

- ¼ teaspoon sea salt or to taste

- ¼ teaspoon chipotle chili powder

- ¼ teaspoon paprika

- ¼ teaspoon cayenne pepper

- ¼ teaspoon chili powder

- ¼ teaspoon pepper

- 1/8 teaspoon garlic powder

- 1 tablespoon olive oil

Toppings: Use any

- Greens of your choice like kale, lettuce, spinach etc.

- Cooked or canned black beans or refried beans

- Salsa

- Guacamole

- Chopped red onion

- Any other toppings of your choice

Directions:

Place a skillet over medium heat. Add oil. When the oil is heated, add tofu, salt and all the spices. Break the tofu simultaneously as it cooks.

Turn off the heat and cool completely.

Divide into meal prep containers. Refrigerate until use. It can last for 10 days.

To serve: Heat thoroughly. Transfer into bowls. Place desired toppings and serve. If using greens, do not place in the meal prep container.

Crispy Quinoa Patties

Ingredients:

- 6 cloves garlic, peeled, minced

- ¼ cup chopped parsley

- Pepper to taste

- Salt to taste

- 2 teaspoons coconut oil

- 4 egg replacers

- 2/3 cup finely diced tomatoes

- 1 cup chopped onions

- 6 cup chopped spinach (bite-size pieces)

- 10 tablespoons gluten-free flour or more if required

- 3 cups cooked quinoa

For yogurt tahini sauce:

- ½ cup vegan yogurt

- ½ teaspoon garlic powder

- 2 teaspoons tahini

- Pepper to taste

- Salt to taste

- Juice of a lime

- 2 teaspoons freshly chopped parsley

- ½ teaspoon extra-virgin olive oil

Serving day ingredients:

- 3 tablespoons coconut oil or more if required

Directions:

To make yogurt tahini sauce: Add all the ingredients for yogurt tahini sauce into a bowl and whisk well. Cover and refrigerate until use.

To make patties: Place a pan over medium heat. Add coconut oil. When the oil is heated, add garlic and onion and cook until onion turns translucent.

Stir in spinach, salt, and pepper and cook until spinach has wilted. Turn off the heat and let it cool for a few minutes. Transfer into a bowl.

Add quinoa, flour, egg replacer, and tomatoes and mix well. If you find the mixture too moist, add some more flour.

Divide the mixture into 20 equal portions and shape into patties.

Place on a tray and refrigerate until use. It can last for 2 days. You can also freeze until firm. Once frozen, transfer into freezer-safe bags. Label the bags with name and date and freeze until use.

To serve: Remove the patties from the refrigerator and thaw completely.

Place a nonstick pan over medium heat. Add a little coconut oil. When the oil is heated, place 4 – 5 patties in the pan. Cook until the underside is golden brown.

Flip sides and cook the other side until golden brown. Remove with a slotted spoon and place on a plate lined with paper towels.

Repeat steps 8 – 9 and make the remaining patties.

Serve with yogurt tahini sauce.

Black Bean & Plantain Arepa Sandwiches

Ingredients:

For plantains:

- ½ tablespoon oil

- 1 large ripe plantains, peeled, cut into ½ inch thick slices, along the diagonal

For black beans:

- ½ can (from a 15 ounces can) black beans, with a little of its liquid

- A pinch salt

- ¼ teaspoon ground cumin

For guacamole:

- 1 ripe avocado, peeled, pitted, mashed

- Salt to taste

- 1 tablespoon chopped cilantro

- 1 – 2 tablespoons lime juice

- 2 tablespoons diced onion

Serving day ingredients:

- 3 large arepas or corn tortillas or pita pockets

- Thinly sliced cabbage

- Hot sauce to taste

- Chopped cilantro

Directions:

Place plantains on a baking sheet lined with parchment paper. Brush oil over the plantains.

Bake in a preheated oven at 425° F for about 20 minutes. Flip sides halfway through baking.

Brush again with some oil. Continue baking until golden brown in color. As the plantains turn light brown, flip the banana slices a couple of times.

Remove from the oven and let it cool completely.

To make black beans: Add black beans, salt and cumin into a pan. Place the pan over medium heat. Heat thoroughly. Turn off the heat and let it cool.

Transfer the banana and black beans into separate airtight containers.

To make guacamole: Add all the ingredients for guacamole into a bowl and mix well. Cover and chill until use.

It can last for 3 days.

To serve: Cut the arepas into 2 halves horizontally. Place bananas, black beans, guacamole, cabbage, hot sauce and cilantro on the bottom half of the arepas. Close with the top of the arepas.

Serve.

Fennel Asparagus Salad

Ingredients:

- 1 medium leek, use only the white part, cut into half-moons

- 1 medium fennel bulb, thinly sliced (about 1 cup)

- 1 ½ tablespoons olive oil

- 2 – 3 large stalks asparagus, sliced

For dressing:

- 1 ½ tablespoons olive oil

- ½ tablespoon minced fresh lemon thyme

- Salt to taste

- ½ teaspoon ground coriander

- 1 tablespoon fresh lemon juice

- Pepper to taste

Serving day ingredients:

- Avocado slices

- 2 tablespoons lightly toasted, chopped almonds

Directions:

Place a pan over medium heat. Add oil. When the oil is heated, add leeks and cook until it wilts and slightly golden at a few spots.

Add salt and stir. Turn off the heat. Transfer into a bowl.

Add asparagus and fennel and toss well.

Add all the ingredients for dressing into a bowl and whisk well. Pour over the salad. Toss well. Refrigerate until use.

It can last for 2 – 3 days.

To serve: Remove from the refrigerator and bring to room temperature.

Top with avocado slices and garnish with almonds. Serve.

Kohlrabi Slaw with Cilantro, Jalapeño and Lime

Ingredients:

- 3 cups sliced kohlrabi (cut into matchsticks)

- ½ teaspoon minced jalapeño or more to taste

- 1 scallion, chopped

- ¼ cup chopped cilantro

- ½ teaspoon grated orange zest

- ½ teaspoon grated lemon zest

- Juice of ½ orange

- Juice of ½ lime

For citrus dressing:

- 2 tablespoons olive oil

- 2 tablespoons fresh orange juice

- 2 tablespoons agave nectar

- ½ tablespoon rice wine vinegar

- 1 ½ tablespoons lime juice or more to taste

- Salt to taste

Directions:

Add all the ingredients for salad into a bowl and toss well.

Add all the ingredients for dressing into another bowl and whisk well. Pour over the salad. Toss well. Cover the bowl.

Refrigerate until use. It can last for 2 days.

Marinated Kale Salad

Ingredients:

For salad:

- 2 bunches curly kale

- 5 tablespoons apple cider vinegar

- 2 tablespoons agave nectar or pure maple syrup

- 2 tablespoons natural almond butter

- 2 – 4 tablespoons tamari or soy sauce or coconut aminos

Optional toppings:

- ½ cup cherry tomatoes

- 2 tablespoons pepitas

- 1 avocado, peeled, pitted, chopped

- Any other toppings of your choice

Directions:

- Dry the kale leaves by patting with a kitchen towel.

- Tear the kale into bite size pieces and place in a large bowl.

- Add rest of the ingredients for salad into a bowl and whisk well.

- Drizzle the dressing over the kale leaves and mix it well using your hands, massaging the leaves lightly.

- Divide into 4 meal prep containers and refrigerate until use. It can last for a day.

Pea Soup

Ingredients:

- 2 onions, chopped

- 2 large potatoes, peeled, cubed

- 6 cups vegetable broth or water

- 2 large cloves garlic, peeled, sliced

- 1.3 pounds peas, fresh or frozen

- 2 tablespoons vegetable oil

- A handful fresh parsley or any other herbs of your choice, chopped

- Salt to taste

- Pepper to taste

Serving day ingredients:

- ½ cup boiled peas

- Vegan yogurt or vegan cream, to drizzle

- Any other toppings of your choice

- 2 tablespoons lemon juice

Directions:

Place a soup pot over medium heat. Add oil. When the oil is heated, add onion and garlic and sauté until pink.

Stir in the stock, salt, pepper, parsley, potatoes and peas. When it begins to boil, lower the heat and cover with a lid. Cook until potatoes are soft. Turn off the heat.

Blend with an immersion blender until smooth. Let it cool completely.

Transfer into an airtight container and refrigerate until use. It can last for 4 days. You can also pour into freezer bags. Label and seal the bags and freeze until use. It can last for 2 months.

To serve: Heat thoroughly. Add lemon juice and stir. Ladle into soup bowls. Garnish with peas, vegan yogurt and any other toppings of your choice and serve.

Avocado Caesar Wraps

Ingredients:

- ½ avocado, peeled, pitted, sliced

- 3 tablespoons vegan Caesar dressing

- 2 tortillas

- 2 big handfuls lettuce, chopped

- ½ can (from a 15 ounces can) chickpeas, rinsed, drained

- ¼ cup chopped cherry tomatoes (optional)

- ¼ cup shredded carrots (optional)

- ½ apple, cored, chopped (optional)

Directions:

Add lettuce into a bowl. Pour dressing over it and stir.

Place tortillas on your countertop. Divide lettuce, chickpeas, tomatoes, carrots, and apples among the tortillas.

Wrap like a burrito. Place in an airtight container. Refrigerate until use. It can last for a day.

Heat in a microwave for a few seconds if desired and serve.

Veggie Coconut Wraps

Ingredients:

- 10 tablespoons hummus

- 1 medium red bell pepper, thinly sliced

- 1 large carrot, shredded

- 2 cups chopped kale

- 4 coconut wraps

- 5 – 6 tablespoons green curry paste

- ¾ cup chopped cilantro

- 1 medium avocado, peeled, pitted, sliced

Directions:

Place the wraps on your countertop.

Mix together hummus and curry paste in a bowl. Divide the mixture equally and spread on the wraps, on the area nearest to you.

Divide the rest of the ingredients equally and place over the wraps in layers.

Start rolling the wraps and place with its seam side facing down, in an airtight container.

Refrigerate until use. It can last for a day.

Cauliflower Soup

Ingredients:

- 2 onions, chopped

- 1 head cauliflower, cut into florets

- 5 – 6 cups vegetable broth

- 8 cloves garlic, peeled, smashed

- 2 tablespoons chopped fresh rosemary or 2 teaspoons dried rosemary

- Salt to taste

- Pepper to taste

Directions:

Place a soup pot over medium heat. Add oil. When the oil is heated, add onion and garlic and sauté until pink. Add a bit of salt and cook until light brown.

Add cauliflower and rosemary and stir for a couple of minutes.

Stir in the stock, salt and pepper. When it begins to boil, lower the heat and cover with a lid. Cook until cauliflower is soft. Turn off the heat.

Blend with an immersion blender until smooth. Let it cool completely.

Transfer into an airtight container and refrigerate until use. It can last for 4 days. You can also pour into freezer bags. Label and seal the bags and freeze until use. It can last for 2 months.

To serve: Heat thoroughly. Ladle into soup bowls. Serve with toppings of your choice.

Spring Vegetables Soup

Ingredients:

- 6 medium carrots, sliced

- 4 large potatoes, sliced

- 1 large onion, chopped

- 6 stalks celery, sliced

- 2 cups peas, fresh or frozen

- Salt to taste

- Pepper to taste

- 4 tablespoons sunflower oil

- 2 vegetable stock cubes

Directions:

Place a soup pot over medium heat. Add oil. When the oil is heated, add onion, carrots, potatoes, celery and peas. Mix well. Cook for 2 – 3 minutes.

Stir in the stock, salt and pepper. When it begins to boil, lower the heat and cover with a lid. Cook until vegetables are soft. Turn off the heat.

Let it cool completely.

Transfer into an airtight container and refrigerate until use. It can last for 4 days. You can also pour into freezer bags. Label and seal the bags and freeze until use. It can last for 2 months.

To serve: Heat thoroughly. Ladle into soup bowls.

Sweet Potato, Lentil & Kale Meal Prep Salads

Ingredients:

- 6 tablespoons brown lentils

- 1 teaspoon olive oil

- 1 medium red bell pepper, diced

- 2 cups cubed sweet potatoes

- 2 heaping cups chopped, curly kale

- 1 small red onion, diced

- Pepper to taste

- Salt to taste

- 1 bay leaf

- 2 tablespoons dried cranberries (optional)

- 2 tablespoons roasted pepitas (pumpkin seeds)

For curry tahini dressing:

- 3 tablespoons tahini

- ¼ teaspoon curry powder or to taste

- 1 tablespoon lemon juice

- 3 – 4 tablespoons water

- 2 small cloves garlic, peeled, minced

Directions:

Place sweet potatoes on a baking sheet. Drizzle oil over it. Sprinkle salt and pepper and mix well. Spread it evenly.

Bake in a preheated oven at 375° F for about 30 minutes or until fork tender. Stir once halfway through baking.

Meanwhile, add lentils into a pan. Pour enough water to cover the lentils by an inch. Add bay leaf and a bit of salt.

When it begins to boil, lower heat and cook until tender. Drain off the excess water.

To make dressing: Add all the ingredients for dressing into a bowl and whisk well.

Place kale in a bowl. Sprinkle some salt and lemon juice over it. Mix well using your hands, simultaneously massaging the kale leaves.

To assemble: Take 2 Mason's jars and add 2 tablespoons dressing in each. Divide the lentils, sweet potatoes, bell pepper, onion and kale among the jars.

Divide the cranberries among the jars. Fasten the lid of the jars and refrigerate until use. It can last for 4 days.

To serve: Transfer the salad into a bowl. Toss well. Sprinkle pumpkin seeds on top if using and serve.

Green Pasta Salad

Ingredients:

- 1 cup cooked, small, tubular pasta

- Olive oil, as required

- 1 cup shredded spinach

- ¼ cup shredded vegan parmesan cheese

- Lemon juice to taste

- 1 cup chopped green beans

- ½ jar basil and olive oil pesto

- Salt to taste

- 2 cloves garlic, peeled, sliced

- 2 tablespoons balsamic vinegar (optional)

- 2 tablespoons olive and basil oil, to drizzle (optional)

Directions:

Drizzle a bit of olive oil over the cooked pasta and toss well.

Place a skillet over medium heat. Add a little olive oil. When the oil is heated, add garlic and green beans and cook until slightly tender. Turn off the heat. Transfer into the bowl of pasta and toss well.

Let it cool completely. Add rest of the ingredients and toss well. Refrigerate until use. It can last for 3 days.

Moroccan Quinoa, Carrot and Chickpea Salad

Ingredients:

For salad:

- 1 cup cooked quinoa

- ½ cup shredded carrots

- 1 cups baby greens of your choice

- 2 tablespoons pumpkin seeds

- ¼ cup chopped parsley

- 2 tablespoons sunflower seeds

- 2 small cloves garlic, peeled, minced

- ½ cup cooked chickpeas

- 2 tablespoons chopped dates

For lemon ginger vinaigrette:

- 2 tablespoons olive oil

- ¼ teaspoon grated fresh ginger

- ¼ teaspoon maple syrup

- 1/8 teaspoon pepper or to taste

- Salt to taste

- ¼ teaspoon ground cinnamon

- 1/8 teaspoon cayenne pepper

- Juice of ½ lemon

Directions:

Divide all the ingredients for salad into 2 meal prep containers. Refrigerate until use. It can last for 3 days.

To make dressing: Add all the ingredients for dressing into a small jar with a lid. Fasten the lid. Shake the jar vigorously until well combined.

To serve: Empty the contents of the meal prep containers into 2 bowls.

Drizzle dressing on top. Toss well and serve.

Serve cold or at room temperature.

Potato Salad

Ingredients:

- 1 pound baby potatoes, rinsed

- ¼ cup chopped, pickled cucumbers

- ½ cup chopped scallions

- 1 ½ cups packed, baby arugula

- 2 tablespoons whole-grain mustard

- ½ teaspoon lightly toasted caraway seeds

- Pepper to taste

- Salt to taste

- 3 teaspoons olive oil

Directions:

Place potatoes in a pot. Pour enough water to cover the potatoes. Place the pot over medium heat. Cook until fork tender.

Drain and place in a bowl. Let it cool completely. Add rest of the ingredients and toss well.

Cover and refrigerate until use. It can last for 2 – 3 days.

Quinoa and Seitan Fajita Bowls

Ingredients:

- 1 cup cooked quinoa

- 2 cloves garlic, peeled, minced

- 6 ounces seitan, sliced

- ¼ cup sliced cherry tomatoes

- 1 tablespoon olive oil

- 1 medium bell pepper of any color, sliced

- ½ cup sliced baby Bella mushrooms

- ¼ teaspoon ground cumin

- 1/8 teaspoon red pepper flakes

- 1/8 teaspoon onion powder

- Pepper to taste

- Salt to taste

- ¼ teaspoon chili powder

- 1/8 teaspoon dried oregano

- 1 cup shredded lettuce

- 1 cup cooked or canned black beans

- 1 teaspoon lime juice or to taste + extra to serve

Directions:

Place a pan over medium-high heat. Add oil. When the oil is heated, add garlic and cook until aromatic.

Stir in the bell pepper, mushrooms, seitan and tomatoes.

Add all the spices into a bowl along with oregano and salt and stir well. Add into the pan and mix well.

Lower heat to medium heat and cook until vegetables are soft.

Stir in the black beans and mix well. Heat thoroughly.

Taste and adjust seasonings if required. Turn off the heat. Cool completely.

Add maple syrup and lime juice into the bowl of quinoa and mix well.

Divide into 2 microwave-safe bowls. Divide the seitan mixture and place over the quinoa.

Cover the bowls with cling wrap and refrigerate until use. It can last for 4 – 5 days.

To serve: Warm in a microwave. Top with some lime juice and serve.

Moroccan Chickpeas

Ingredients:

- 2 cans (15 ounces each) chickpeas, drained, rinsed

- 2 bell peppers, chopped

- 2 onions, chopped

- 2 cans (19 ounces each) diced tomatoes with its juices

- 4 cups cubed sweet potato (½ inch cubes)

- 3 tablespoons Moroccan spice blend

- Vegetable broth or water, if required

Serving day ingredients:

- Chopped parsley

- Lemon juice

Directions:

Place a skillet over medium heat. Add all the ingredients into the skillet and mix well. Sprinkle some water or broth.

Cover and cook for 30-40 minutes or until sweet potatoes are tender. Add more water or stock if the mixture is getting stuck to the bottom of the pan.

Turn off the heat and cool completely. Transfer into an airtight container and refrigerate until use. It can last for 4 days.

To freeze: Transfer into freezer-safe bags. Squeeze the bags to remove any air that is present. Seal and label the bags with name and date. Freeze until use. It can last for 3 months.

To serve: Remove from the refrigerator or freezer and thaw completely.

Transfer into a skillet and heat thoroughly. Sprinkle some water or broth while heating.

Sesame Tofu Quinoa Bowls

Ingredients:

- ½ pound green beans, trimmed, halved

- 2 cups broccoli florets

- ½ block extra-firm tofu, pressed of excess moisture

- 1 cup cooked quinoa

For dressing:

- 2 tablespoons toasted sesame oil

- ½ teaspoon arrowroot or tapioca starch or cornstarch

- ¼ teaspoon ground ginger

- ¼ teaspoon garlic powder

- 1 tablespoon tamari

- Crushed red pepper flakes to taste

- Salt to taste

To garnish:

- Black sesame seeds

Directions:

Spread the green beans on 1/3 part of a baking sheet. Spread tofu on another 1/3 portion and broccoli florets on 1/3 of the portion of the baking sheet.

Add all the ingredients for dressing into a bowl and whisk well. Drizzle over the beans, broccoli and tofu. Mix each of them.

Bake in a preheated oven at 375° F for about 30 minutes. Stir once halfway through baking.

Remove from the oven and cool completely.

Divide into 2 meal prep containers. Also divide the quinoa among the containers.

Refrigerate until use. It can last for 3 days. Top with tamari or some hot sauce.

Portobello Fajita Meal Prep Bowls

Ingredients:

For spice blend:

- ½ teaspoon garlic powder

- ½ teaspoon ground cumin

- ½ teaspoon red pepper flakes

- ½ teaspoon onion powder

- ½ teaspoon chili powder

- ½ teaspoon salt

For fajita bowls:

- 6 tablespoons quinoa

- 2 Portobello mushrooms, cut into strips

- ½ zucchini, sliced

- 1 tablespoon olive oil

- 1 bell pepper, deseed if desired, sliced

- 1 small red onion, sliced

Other ingredients:

- 2 lime wedges

- ½ cup black beans

Serving day ingredients:

- Avocado slices

- Salsa

- Vegan yogurt etc.

Directions:

To make spice blend: Add all the ingredients for spice blend into a bowl and stir.

Add half the spice blend mixture and cook the quinoa following the instructions on the package. Once cooked, set aside to cool.

Add all the vegetables into a baking dish. Drizzle oil over it. Sprinkle remaining spice blend mixture and toss well.

Bake in a preheated oven at 425° F for about 20 minutes. Stir once halfway through baking. Remove from the oven and cool completely.

Divide the quinoa into 2 meal prep containers. Layer with vegetables and black beans. Refrigerate until use. It can last for 5 days.

To serve: Heat if desired. Serve with the suggested serving options or with any other toppings of your choice.

Low carbohydrate sausage rolls

Ingredients:

4 hot dogs

120 g grated mozzarella

75 g almond flour

1 tsp xanthan gum

2 tbsp cream cheese

2 medium eggs

4 tbsp seeds & kernel mix (sesame seeds, poppy seeds, linseed)

1 - 2 tsp onion powder

1 tsp garlic powder

Directions

Put the grated mozzarella and cream cheese in a microwave-proof bowl and heat in the microwave for 1.5 minutes, until the cheese has melted. Mix everything well and set aside.

In another bowl, mix the almond flour, 1 egg and the xanthan gum. Add the cheese mix to the flour mix and knead with wet hands into a lump-free batter.

Shape the dough into 4 equally sized balls and places them on a baking sheet with a sheet of baking paper. Carefully roll out each ball with wet hands until they are approximately 40 cm long.

Then wrap each piece of dough tightly around a hot dog and place them on a plate. Then whisk the remaining egg in a bowl with a whisk and spread it over the hot dogs with a brush. Then mix all seeds and herbs in a bowl and dip the hot dogs in the spice mixture.

Put the hot dogs back on the baking tray and bake for 20 minutes in the preheated oven until golden brown. Enjoy your meal!

Low-carbohydrate salad nicoise

Ingredients:

Salad:

1 large can of tuna in water

1 tbsp mayonnaise

150 gr haricots verts

2 eggs (M or L)

150 g romaine lettuce

30 g sliced red onion

1/2 red pepper

salt and pepper to taste

Dressing:

40 ml of olive oil

1 tbsp mustard

1 tbsp white wine vinegar

1 tbsp lemon juice

Directions

Bring a pan of water to be boiled. Add the eggs to the pan and cook for 6 to 8 minutes. Then grab another pan and fill it with water. Add the haricots verts to the pan and bring to the boil. Cook the haricots verts until al dente within 4-6 minutes. After cooking, drain the water from the pan well.

Meanwhile, drain the tuna can and mix the tuna pieces in a bowl with the mayonnaise, salt, and pepper. Then cut the red onion and bell pepper into small strips.

Then make the dressing by mixing the olive oil, white wine vinegar, mustard, and lemon juice. After cooking, scare the eggs in cold water. Peel the eggs and cut the eggs into smaller pieces.

Then divide the romaine lettuce over two plates and add the red onion, pepper, tuna, and haricots verts. Finally, sprinkle the niçoise salad with the mustard dressing. Enjoy your meal!

Low-carbohydrate pumpkin soup

Ingredients:

400 g pumpkin (cubes)

2 tomatoes

1 onion

1 leek

1 clove of garlic, crushed

100 ml of cooking cream

700 ml of water

1 vegetable stock cube

125 gr sour cream

parsley to taste

Salt and pepper to taste.

1 tbsp olive oil or butter

Directions

Dice the pumpkin, onion, leek, and tomatoes on a large cutting board. Take a large soup pot and heat in it a tbsp of butter or olive oil. Put garlic and onions in the pan and fry for 1-2 minutes, until the onion starts to discolor. Then add the remains of the vegetables and fry for 3 minutes while stirring.

Add the water to the pan and crumble the stock cube over the pan. Bring the contents of the pan to be boiled and cook for 20 minutes over low heat.

Remove the pan from the heat after 20 minutes and puree the contents of the pan with a blender to a smooth soup. Then add the cream and cook for 2 minutes. Taste the soup and season with a little salt and pepper if necessary.

Divide the soup into four soup bowls, garnish with parsley, and scoop in each bowl and sour cream. Enjoy your meal!

Chapter 13: Dinner Recipes

Baked avocado wrapped in bacon

Ingredients:

2 avocados

8 slices of bacon

50 g of grated cheese of your choice

Directions

Preheat the oven to 200 degrees and layout a baking sheet with some baking paper.

Cut avocados in half; remove seeds, and then peel.

Fill two halves with cheese and then cover with the other half.

Wrap each avocado with four slices of bacon.

Put the avocados on the baking tray and bake for about 8-15 minutes until crispy.

Remove avocado from the oven, cut open, and serve immediately. Good Appetite!

Spicy Shrimp Kebabs

Ingredients:

500 g shrimp

2 tbsp olive oil, native

Sea salt and cayenne pepper

1 teaspoon paprika powder

1 teaspoon garlic powder

1 teaspoon onion powder

1 teaspoon oregano, dried

2 lemons, sliced

Directions

Preheat oven to 180 degrees.

Put salt, cayenne pepper, paprika, garlic powder, onion powder and oregano in a small bowl and mix.

Put the shrimp with the olive oil in a bowl.

Add the spice mixture and cover the shrimp evenly.

Put shrimp together with the slices of lemon on wooden skewers.

Put the skewers in the oven for 10-15 minutes and turn occasionally.

Tofu Setan (soy)

INGREDIENTS:

1 12-oz. pack extra firm tofu (drained, cubed)

2 tbsp. coconut oil

2 garlic cloves

1 medium onion (chopped)

2 red chilis (finely chopped, more to taste)

2 tbsp. soy sauce

1½ tbsp. low-carb maple syrup

½ tbsp. mustard

¼ cup water

Optional: ¼ cup spring onions (finely chopped)

DIRECTIONS

Take a large skillet and put it over medium-high heat.

Add the coconut oil and tofu cubes, stirring occasionally, until the tofu starts to brown.

Meanwhile, in a blender or food processor, add the garlic, onions, chilis, soy sauce, maple syrup, and mustard; process the ingredients into a rough paste.

Add the paste to the skillet and stir for about a minute or until the paste starts to caramelize.

Add the water to the skillet and turn the heat down to medium.

Let the tofu setan cook while occasionally stirring, until most of the water has evaporated.

Take the skillet off the heat and allow the tofu setan to cool down for a minute.

Garnish with the optional spring onions if desired, serve, and enjoy!

Alternatively, store the tofu setan in an airtight container in the fridge. Consume within 3 days. Store in the freezer for a maximum of 30 days and thaw at room temperature. Use a microwave, toaster oven, or frying pan to reheat the tofu setan.

Moo Goo Gai Pan (soy)

INGREDIENTS:

1 12-oz. pack extra firm tofu (drained, cubed)

2 tbsp. coconut oil

½ cup carrots (julienned or thinly sliced)

2 cups mushrooms (sliced)

1 cup bamboo shoots

1 tbsp. water

2 garlic cloves (minced)

1-inch piece ginger (finely minced)

Salt and pepper to taste

Sauce:

1 cup vegetable broth (*see recipe*)

1 tbsp. low-carb maple syrup

1 tbsp. low-sodium soy sauce

1 tbsp. sesame oil

1 tsp. agar

DIRECTIONS

Take a large skillet, put it over medium-high heat and add 1 tablespoon of the coconut oil.

Add the carrots and a tablespoon of water. Cook the carrots for 3 minutes while stirring.

Add in the mushrooms and cook until the slices are lightly brown and tender.

Stir in the bamboo shoots and cook all ingredients for about a minute. Add salt and pepper to taste.

Remove the vegetables from the skillet, transfer them onto a plate, and cover with foil to keep the veggies warm.

In a small bowl, mix the sauce ingredients. Stir well and set the sauce aside.

Wipe the skillet with a paper towel to remove any excess liquid and add the remaining tablespoon of coconut oil to the skillet.

Add the tofu cubes to the skillet and stir while seasoning the tofu cubes with salt and pepper to taste.

Continue to add the ginger and garlic to the skillet. Allow the ingredients to cook for about a minute.

Add the vegetables back into the skillet, heat them through for a minute, and then pour in the previously made sauce.

Turn heat up to high and wait until the sauce begins to boil. Allow it to cook for a minute while occasionally stirring.

Take the skillet of the heat, serve, and enjoy!

Alternatively, store the moo goo gai pan in an airtight container in the fridge. Consume within 3 days. Store in the freezer for a maximum of 30 days, and thaw at room temperature. Use a microwave, toaster oven or skillet to reheat the moo goo gai pan.

Cashew Siam Stir-Fry (soy, nuts)

INGREDIENTS:

2 tbsp. olive oil

½ cup raw cashews (unsalted)

½ green onion (finely chopped)

4 garlic cloves (minced)

1-inch piece ginger (grated)

1 red bell pepper (seeded, chopped)

1 (10 oz. pack) extra firm tofu (drained, cubed)

1 tsp. chili flakes

Sauce:

1 tbsp. low-sodium soy sauce

3 tsp. rice vinegar

1 tbsp. low-carb maple syrup

¼ cup vegetable broth (*see recipe*, or use water)

1 tsp. sesame oil

Total number of ingredients: 13

DIRECTIONS

Put the olive oil in a large skillet over medium heat.

Add the cashews to the skillet and stir fry for 2 minutes.

Stir the chopped onion and garlic into the skillet. Keep stirring while cooking until the onion is translucent. This should take about two minutes.

Add the ginger and chopped bell pepper. Increase the heat to medium-high and cook the ingredients for about 3 minutes while stirring.

Add the tofu cubes and chili flakes. Cook for another 3 minutes, stirring occasionally.

Mix the sauce ingredients in a medium-sized bowl until no lumps remain and add it to the skillet.

Stir and cook all ingredients together for another minute, then bring the heat down to a simmer while stirring occasionally until the sauce starts to thicken.

Take the skillet off the heat, divide the cashew stir-fry between 2 bowls, serve and enjoy!

Alternatively, store the cashew stir-fry in an airtight container in the fridge and consume within 3 days. Store in the freezer for a maximum of 30 days and thaw at room temperature. Use a microwave or pot to reheat the cashew stir-fry.

Vegan Chili with Vegan Sausage

Ingredients:

- 1 tablespoon olive oil

- ½ cup chopped red bell pepper

- 1 cup chopped kale

- ½ cup chopped onion

- ½ tablespoon chopped garlic

- ½ package (from a 12.95 ounces package) vegan sausage, chopped

- ¼ cup white wine

- 1 cup chopped tomato

- Freshly ground pepper to taste

- ½ teaspoon dried ground sage

- 3 cups vegetable stock

- 1 can (15 ounces) unsalted kidney beans, rinsed, drained, divided

- 1 ½ cans (15 ounces each) cannellini beans, rinsed, drained, divided

- ½ teaspoon salt or to taste

- ½ teaspoon crushed red pepper

Directions

Place a Dutch oven over medium-high heat. Add oil. When the oil is heated, add onions, garlic, sausage and bell pepper. Sauté for 3-4 minutes.

Stir in the tomatoes, spices, wine, salt and sage. Cook until the wine reduces to half its original quantity.

Add stock and stir. Add ½ can kidney beans and ¾ can cannellini beans into a bowl and mash with a potato masher. Add into the pot. Also add the remaining beans. Let it simmer for 5-8 minutes.

Add kale and cook until it wilts. Add oregano and stir. Taste and adjust the seasoning if required. Turn off the heat and cool completely.

Transfer into an airtight container and refrigerate until use. It can last for 4 days. To freeze: Transfer into freezer bags and freeze until use. It can last for 3 months.

Vegetable Chili

Ingredients:

- 4 tablespoons olive oil

- 1 large red bell pepper, chopped

- 2 onions, chopped

- 2 large cloves garlic, finely chopped

- 2 small zucchinis, trimmed, diced

- 2 ears corn, use the kernels

- 2 small yellow squashes, diced

- 4 cans (10 ounces each) diced tomatoes with green chilies

- 3 cups cooked or canned kidney beans, rinsed

- 3 cups cooked or canned black beans, rinsed

- 4 tablespoons tomato paste

- 2 tablespoons chili powder

- 4 teaspoons dried oregano

- 4 teaspoons ground cumin

- Cayenne pepper to taste

- Salt to taste

- Pepper to taste

Directions:

Place a Dutch oven over medium-high heat. Add oil. When the oil is heated, add onions and sauté until translucent. Add garlic, spices and oregano. Sauté for few seconds until aromatic.

Add the vegetables and cook until tender.

Stir in the rest of the ingredients and bring to a boil.

Lower heat and cook for about 20 minutes. Taste and adjust seasonings if required. Turn off the heat and cool completely.

Transfer into an airtight container and refrigerate until use. It can last for 4 days. To freeze: Transfer into freezer bags and freeze until use. It can last for 3 months.

Tempeh Taco Salad Bowls

Ingredients:

For tempeh taco meat:

- 2 packages (8 ounces each) tempeh, crumbled

- 3 tablespoons chili powder

- ½ cup canned tomato sauce

- 2 tablespoons olive oil or avocado oil

- 5 teaspoons taco seasoning or to taste

- Salt to taste

- Pepper to taste

For bowls:

- 12 cup chopped romaine lettuce

- ½ cup chopped red onion

- 2 cups diced cherry tomatoes

- ¼ cup chopped fresh cilantro

- 1 ½ cups cooked black beans

- 2 avocados, peeled, pitted sliced

- Salt to taste

Serving day ingredients:

- 3 lime wedges

- Fresh salsa

- Tortilla chips

- Hot sauce

Directions:

Place a large skillet over medium-high heat. Add oil. When the oil is heated, add tempeh and cook for 4 – 5 minutes.

Add rest of the ingredients and mix well. Cook until nearly dry. Turn off the heat and let it cool.

Add tomatoes, cilantro, onion, and salt into a bowl and toss well.

Take 6 meal prep containers. Divide the lettuce, tomato mixture, tempeh, and black beans among the containers.

Close the lid and refrigerate until use. It can last 4-5 days.

Thaw completely before serving. Serve with avocado, lime wedges, salsa, hot sauce and tortilla chips.

BBQ-Flavored Seitan and Avocado Wraps

Ingredients:

- 16 ounces seitan, drained, finely diced

- 4 wraps (10 – 12 inches each)

- 1 cup vegan BBQ sauce

- 4 tablespoons hemp seeds (optional)

- 1 avocado, peeled, pitted, thinly sliced

- Vegan mayonnaise or mustard (or use both), as required

- Greens of your choice

- 2 tomatoes, thinly sliced

- 1 avocado, peeled, pitted, thinly sliced

Directions:

Place a skillet over medium heat. Add BBQ sauce and seitan and mix well. Heat thoroughly and cook until nearly dry.

Spread the wraps on your countertop. Smear vegan mayonnaise or mustard or a little of both.

Scatter hemp seeds if using. Spread some greens along the diameter of the wraps.

Divide the seitan and place over the greens, along the center. Place avocados on one side and tomatoes on the other side of the seitan.

Wrap tightly and place in an airtight container.

It can last for a day.

To serve: Heat in a microwave for 20 – 30 seconds and serve.

Mushroom, Spinach, and Cheddar Wraps

Ingredients:

- 5 ounces white or cremini or baby mushrooms

- 2 wraps or flour tortillas (10 inches each)

- Salsa, as required (optional)

- 5 ounces fresh baby spinach

- ½ cup grated non-dairy cheddar cheese

Directions:

Place a skillet over medium heat. Add mushrooms. Sprinkle a little water and cook until mushrooms are tender.

Add spinach and cook until it wilts. Discard cooked water if any.

Place wraps on your countertop. Divide equally the mixture among the wraps. Drizzle some salsa on top. Wrap and place in an airtight container with the seam side facing down.

To serve: Heat for 20 – 30 seconds in the microwave and serve.

Vegan Tuna Lemon Pasta

Ingredients:

- 4 servings cooked pasta of your choice

- 4 tablespoons olive oil

- 2 packets vegan tuna (Like Good Catch Foods Tuna)

- ½ cup chopped fresh parsley

- ½ cup cooked pasta water

- 6 large cloves garlic, pressed

- Juice of a large lemon

Directions:

Place a large pan over medium heat. Add oil. When the oil is heated, add garlic and cook until brown.

Raise the heat to high heat and add vegan tuna. Break with a fork as it cooks. Add lemon and mix well. Lower the heat and add pasta. Toss well. Add the pasta water and mix well. Turn off the heat.

When it cools, transfer into an airtight container. Refrigerate until use. It can last for 2 days.

To serve: Heat thoroughly. Add parsley and toss well. Serve.

Veggie Salad Jars

Ingredients:

For salad:

- 1 tomato, chopped

- ½ courgette, sliced

- 1 medium eggplant, sliced

- 1 small cucumber, deseeded, chopped

- 3.5 ounces vegan feta cheese, crumbled

- ½ tablespoon olive oil

- 1.7 ounces kalamata olives

- 4.5 ounces canned or cooked chickpeas

- A handful of mint leaves, torn or chopped

- ½ yellow bell pepper, deseeded, chopped

- 0.8 ounce sundried tomatoes

- A handful of dill leaves, chopped

- Salt to taste

- Pepper to taste

For pickled onion dressing:

- ½ red onion, thinly sliced

- 2 tablespoons white wine vinegar

- 3 ½ tablespoons extra-virgin olive oil

- ¼ teaspoon coriander seeds

- 2 tablespoons lemon juice

- Water, as required

- Salt to taste

- Pepper to taste

Directions:

To make pickled onion dressing: Add vinegar, onions, coriander seeds, and 3-4 tablespoons water dressing into a small pan. Place the pan over medium-low heat. Cook until the onions are translucent.

Turn off heat and set aside to cool. Add lemon juice and oil into the pickled onion Add salt and pepper and stir.

Brush eggplant and courgette slices with olive oil.

Place a griddle pan over medium-high heat. When the pan begins to smoke, place eggplant and courgette slices on it.

Cook until the underside is slightly charred. Flip sides and cook the other side until slightly charred. Remove onto a plate. Sprinkle salt and pepper and set aside.

Divide the pickled onion into 4 mason's jars.

Divide and layer with tomatoes, vegan feta cheese, chickpeas and olives in the jars. Press slightly with a spoon to push the salad.

Layer with sundried tomatoes along with a little of its oil followed by the cooked vegetables. Next layer will be cucumber, followed by bell pepper, mint and dill leaves.

Fasten the lid and refrigerate until use. It can last for 2 days.

To serve: Empty the jars into individual serving bowls. Toss well and serve.

Buffalo Chickpea Pita Pockets with Creamy Avocado

Ingredients:

- ½ can (from a 15 ounces can) chickpeas

- ½ tablespoon coconut oil

- 2 tablespoons unsweetened almond milk

- 2 pita rounds, to serve

- 1 medium cucumber, peeled, chopped

- 2 tablespoons Buffalo hot sauce

- ½ ripe avocado, peeled, pitted, chopped

- 1 tablespoon lemon juice

- A handful kale leaves, torn

Directions:

Add chickpeas, buffalo sauce and coconut oil into a baking dish. Mix well.

Bake in a preheated oven at 400° F for about 15 minutes. Stir a couple of times while baking. Remove from the oven and let it cool. Transfer into an airtight container. Refrigerate until use.

Meanwhile, add avocado, almond milk, salt and lemon juice into a blender and blend until creamy.

Pour into a bowl. Cover and chill until use. It can last for 2 days.

To serve: Heat chickpeas and fill the pita pockets with it. Place kale and cucumber. Spoon some avocado sauce and serve.

Baked Ziti

Ingredients:

- 1 pound dried pasta

- 20 basil leaves, torn + extra to garnish

- Salt to taste

- Pepper to taste

- 2 jars (24 ounces each) marinara sauce

- 16 ounces vegan mozzarella cheese, diced

- Boiling water, as required

Directions:

Place pasta in a large bowl. Add boiling water into the bowl such that the pasta is covered with water (about 2 inches above the pasta). Set aside for 45 minutes. Drain excess water.

Add marinara sauce and basil leaves into a baking dish and mix well.

Add 12 ounces mozzarella cheese and toss well. Scatter the remaining cheese on top.

Cover the dish with foil and refrigerate until use. It can last for 2 days.

To serve: Bake covered, in a preheated oven at 350° F for about 45 minutes. Uncover and bake for 15 minutes.

Let it sit on the countertop for 15 minutes. Garnish with basil and serve.

Lentil Balls with Zesty Rice

Ingredients:

For lentil balls:

- 1 can (15 ounces) brown or black lentils, drained, rinsed

- 1 ½ tablespoons chopped, dried mushrooms

- 1 ½ tablespoons tomato paste

- ¼ teaspoon pepper or to taste

- ½ cup walnut halves

- 2 teaspoons tomato paste

- ¼ cup vegan breadcrumbs

- A handful fresh parsley, chopped

For zesty rice:

- ½ cup + 1/3 cup water

- 1 tablespoon lemon juice

- 1 teaspoon grated lemon zest

- 2/3 cup uncooked basmati rice

- A handful fresh parsley, minced

- Salt to taste

For toppings:

- 1 cup chopped lettuce

- 1 small onion, thinly sliced

- ½ cup halved cherry tomatoes

- 2 lemon wedges

Directions:

For lentil balls: Add lentils, mushrooms, parsley, pepper, salt, tomato paste and walnuts into the food processor bowl. Pulse until chopped into smaller pieces. Do not over process.

Add into a bowl. Add breadcrumbs and mix well.

Scoop out about 2 tablespoons of the mixture and shape into a ball. Repeat this step and make the remaining balls.

Place the balls on a lined baking sheet.

Bake in a preheated oven at 375° F for about 20 minutes. Flip sides halfway through baking.

Remove from the oven and cool completely.

To make zesty rice: Add water and rice into a saucepan. Place the saucepan over medium flame. When it begins to boil, lower the heat and cover with a lid. Cook until dry. Turn off the heat and cool completely.

Transfer the rice and lentil balls into meal prep containers. Refrigerate until use. It can last for 3 – 4 days.

To serve: Heat thoroughly the rice and lentil balls.

Add lettuce, onion and tomatoes into a bowl and toss well. Divide into 2 serving plates. Layer with rice. Place lentil balls on top. Serve with lemon wedges.

Butternut Squash Enchiladas

Ingredients:

For enchiladas:

- 1 cup pureed, roasted butternut squash – procedure given in the directions

- 1 small jalapeño, deseeded, minced

- ½ cup thinly sliced Brussels sprouts

- ½ teaspoon chili powder

- Salt to taste

- 12 ounces mild salsa Verde

- ½ small red onion, finely chopped

- 1 – 2 cloves garlic, peeled, minced

- ½ teaspoon ground cumin

- 1/8 teaspoon cayenne pepper

- ½ can (from a 15 ounces can) black beans, drained, rinsed

- 6 corn tortillas

- ½ tablespoon extra-virgin olive oil

For cashew sour cream:

- ½ cup cashews, soaked in water for an hour

- Juice of ½ lemon

- ¼ cup water

- Salt to taste

For topping:

- A handful fresh cilantro, chopped

- 1 tablespoon pumpkin seeds

Directions:

Place a sheet of parchment paper over a baking sheet. Take a small butternut squash. Cut into 2 halves. Discard the seeds and membrane. Brush with oil and place on the baking sheet.

Roast in a preheated oven at 400° F for about 45 minutes.

Remove from the oven and let it cool. Scoop out the pulp from the squash and measure out 1 cup. Add into a bowl.

Place a skillet over medium heat. Add ½ tablespoon oil. When the oil is heated, add onion and cook until pink.

Stir in the garlic and jalapeño and cook for a couple of minutes.

Add Brussels sprouts, spices and salt. Sauté until slightly soft. Stir in the black beans. Turn off the heat. Let it cool completely. Transfer into the bowl of butternut squash. Mix well.

Spread a thin layer of salsa on the bottom of a baking dish (8 x 8 inches).

Spread the tortillas on your countertop. Place 1/3 cup of butternut squash mixture onto each tortilla, along the diameter.

Place the rolled tortillas in the baking dish, with the seam side facing down.

Drizzle the remaining salsa over the enchiladas. Spread the salsa evenly.

Cover the dish and refrigerate until use. Use within a day.

To make cashew sour cream: Add all the ingredients for cashew sour cream into a blender and blend until smooth. Pour into a bowl. Cover and chill until use.

Remove the dish and the cashew sour cream from the refrigerator 30 minutes before baking.

Bake in a preheated oven at 375° F for about 20 to 30 minutes.

Remove from the oven and cool for a while. Drizzle cashew sour cream on top. Garnish with pumpkin seeds and cilantro and serve.

Plantain Black Bean Enchilada Bake

Ingredients:

For plantains:

- 1 tablespoon coconut oil, melted

- 2 large ripe plantains, peeled, cut into slices lengthwise (10 slices in all)

For black beans:

- 1 can (15 ounces) black beans, drained

- Salt to taste

- 1 teaspoon ground cumin

For cheese sauce:

- ½ cup + 2 tablespoons cashews

- ¼ teaspoon sea salt or to taste

- ¼ teaspoon ground cumin

- Warm water, to blend, as required

- 2 tablespoons nutritional yeast

- 1/8 teaspoon garlic powder

- ¼ small chipotle chili in adobo sauce or more to taste (optional)

For enchilada sauce:

- 1 cup +1 ½ tablespoons vegetable broth

- 2 cloves garlic, peeled, smashed

- ½ cup chopped onion

- 3 dried chilies, like ancho chili

- 1 dried arbol chilies

- ½ cup water

- 2 tablespoons tomato paste

- ½ teaspoon ground smoked paprika

- ½ teaspoon dried oregano

- ½ teaspoon ground cumin

- ¼ teaspoon salt

Toppings:

- Chopped cilantro

- 1 small red onion, chopped

- 1 jalapeño, chopped

- Guacamole or avocado slices

Directions:

To make enchilada sauce: Place a skillet over medium heat. Add 1 ½ tablespoons broth, garlic, and onion and sauté until lightly brown.

Stir in the dried chilies and sauté for a couple of minutes. Stir in water and remaining broth. When it begins to boil, lower the heat and cover with a lid. Cook for 10 – 12 minutes.

Add tomato paste, salt, oregano, and spices and mix well. Cover and continue cooking for another 5 minutes. Turn off the heat.

Add into a blender. Blend until smooth. Taste and adjust the salt if necessary.

Use about a cup. Store leftovers in an airtight container in the refrigerator.

Place plantain slices on a lined baking sheet. Do not overlap. Brush with oil on top. Flip sides and brush with oil on the other side as well.

Bake in a preheated oven at 425° F for about 30 minutes or until golden brown. Flip sides halfway through baking.

To make black beans: Add all the ingredients for black beans into a saucepan. Place the saucepan over medium heat. Mix well. Heat thoroughly. Remove from heat.

To make cheese sauce: Add all the ingredients for cheese sauce into a blender and blend until smooth. Taste and adjust the seasonings or nutritional yeast if required.

To assemble: Spread a little of the enchilada sauce on the bottom of a baking dish.

Place a layer of bananas. Spread a layer of cheese sauce. Spread half the beans. Spread some good amount of enchilada sauce. Place another layer of plantain slices.

Spread some more of the cheese sauce over the plantains. Spread the remaining beans over the plantains. Spread remaining enchilada sauce. Spread any remaining cheese sauce.

Cover the dish with foil. Refrigerate until use. Use within 4 - 5 days. You can also freeze it for a month.

Bake in a preheated oven at 350° F for about 30 minutes.

Serve with suggested serving options.

Seitan Stew

Ingredients:

- 6 guajillo chilies, discard stems and seeds, chopped into large pieces

- 4 dried chilies de Abrol, discard stems and seeds, chopped into large pieces

- 8 dried New Mexico chilies, discard stems and seeds, chopped into large pieces

- 8 cups vegetable broth, divided

- 4 tablespoons olive oil

- 6 cloves garlic, minced

- 4 teaspoons dried oregano

- 3 tablespoons apple cider vinegar

- 4 tablespoons masa harina

- 2 pounds seitan, chopped

- 16 ounces waxy potatoes, chopped into cubes

- Salt to taste

- 3 cups fire-roasted, canned, chopped tomatoes

- 1 onion, chopped

- 2 tablespoons ground cumin

- ½ teaspoon pepper or to taste

- 2 tablespoons soy sauce

Directions

Place a pan over medium heat. When the pan heats, add all the chilies and cook for a couple of minutes until slightly soft.

Transfer into a microwavable bowl. Add 4 cups water. Cover and cook on high for 3 minutes. Remove from the microwave and add into a blender. Also add the tomatoes and blend until smooth.

Place a soup pot over medium heat. Add 2 tablespoons of oil. Add onion and a bit of salt and cook until pink. Stir in the garlic and cook for a few seconds until aromatic.

Stir in the oregano and cumin. Cook for a few seconds stirring constantly until aromatic. Stir in the blended mixture, rest of the broth and potatoes. When it begins to boil, lower the heat and cover with a lid. Cook until potatoes are soft.

Meanwhile, place a pan over medium heat. Add remaining oil. When the oil is heated, add seitan and sauté for a few minutes, until light brown. Remove onto a plate and set aside.

Place masa harina in a bowl. Add a little of the soup and mix well. Pour it back into the pot. Also add in the vinegar, soy sauce and seitan and stir constantly until thick. Add salt and pepper to taste. Turn off the heat and cool completely.

Transfer into an airtight container and refrigerate until use. It can last for 4 -5 days.

To serve: Heat thoroughly. Ladle into soup bowls and serve.

Smoky Tempeh Tostadas with Mango Cabbage Slaw

Ingredients:

For tempeh:

- 2 packages (8 ounces each) tempeh, cut into thin pieces

- 2 teaspoons chili powder

- 1 teaspoon ground cumin

- 1 teaspoon garlic powder

- ½ teaspoon pepper

- 1 teaspoon onion powder

- Oil, as required

- ½ cup soy sauce or tamari

- Hot sauce to taste

- 1 teaspoon liquid smoke

For mango cabbage slaw:

- 3 cups shredded red cabbage

- 1 cup chopped cilantro

- 1 ½ cups diced mango

- 2 tablespoons fresh lime juice

- 2 teaspoons agave nectar

- 2 teaspoons apple cider vinegar

Serving day ingredients:

- 12 corn tortillas

- Chopped cilantro

- Chopped avocado

- Salsa

Directions:

To make tempeh: Add soy sauce, hot sauce, liquid smoke and spices into a bowl and mix until well combined.

Add tempeh and stir until well coated with the mixture. Let it marinate for 10 minutes.

Place a skillet over medium heat. Add some oil. When the oil is heated, add tempeh and cook until the underside is brown. Flip sides and cook the other side until brown. Remove with a slotted spoon and place on a plate. Let it cool completely.

To make slaw: Add all the ingredients for slaw into a bowl and toss well.

Transfer the slaw and tempeh into meal prep containers. Refrigerate until use. It can last for 3 days.

To serve: Place corn tortillas on a baking sheet. Bake in a preheated oven at 400° F for about 10 minutes or until golden brown.

Heat the tempeh. Add salt to slaw and toss well.

Divide the tempeh among the tortillas. Place slaw on top. Place the suggested toppings and serve.

Curried Cauliflower & Chickpea Burritos

Ingredients:

For coconut basmati rice:

- ½ cup water

- ½ cup basmati rice

- ½ cup light coconut milk

- Salt to taste

For curried cauliflower and chickpeas:

- ½ tablespoon vegetable oil

- 2 cloves garlic, peeled, minced

- ½ tablespoon garam masala

- 1 ½ cups small cauliflower florets

- ¼ cup water

- 1 tablespoon tomato paste

- Salt to taste

- Pepper to taste

- ½ onion, diced

- 1 teaspoon freshly grated ginger

- ½ teaspoon ground cumin

- ½ can (from a 14 ounces can) diced tomatoes

- ½ can (from a 14 ounces can) chickpeas, drained, rinsed

- 2 tablespoons chopped cilantro

To assemble:

- 2 large or 3 medium flour tortillas

Directions:

To make coconut basmati rice: Add water and coconut milk into a saucepan. Place the saucepan over high heat. When it begins to boil, add the rice and stir. Lower the heat. Cover and cook until dry. Turn off the heat. Let it rest for 5 minutes.

Add salt and fluff with a fork.

To make curried cauliflower and chickpeas: Place a skillet over medium heat. Add oil. When the oil is heated, add onion and cook until translucent. Stir in the ginger, garlic, cumin and garam masala and sauté for a few seconds until aromatic.

Stir in the tomatoes, cauliflower and water. Mix well. Cover with a lid. Lower the heat and simmer until cauliflower is tender.

Add tomato paste and chickpeas and cook uncovered until thick. Stir occasionally.

Turn off the heat. Add cilantro, salt and pepper and mix well.

Place the tortillas on your countertop. Divide the rice among the tortillas and spread on the center. Spread cauliflower and chickpeas. Over the rice. Wrap like a burrito.

Place in an airtight container and refrigerate until use. It can last for a day.

Teriyaki Setian with Mashed Kabocha

Ingredients:

For teriyaki sauce:

- 4 tablespoons soy sauce

- 2 tablespoons orange juice

- 2 tablespoons brown sugar

- ½ teaspoon sesame oil

- ¼ teaspoon red pepper flakes or to taste

- 1 clove garlic, minced

- ½ tablespoon cornstarch

- 2 tablespoons water

- Salt to taste

- 1 teaspoon minced ginger

- 1 ½ tablespoons rice vinegar

For seitan:

- 4 ounces seitan, sliced

- ¼ pound winter squash, peeled, cubed

- ¾ cup broccoli florets

- ½ tablespoon sesame seeds

- Salt to taste

Directions:

To make teriyaki sauce: Add all the ingredients for the sauce into a saucepan and whisk well.

Place the saucepan over medium heat. Stir constantly until thick. Turn off the heat.

Steam the broccoli and winter squash until tender.

Place a nonstick pan over medium-high heat. Add seitan and cook until the underside is golden brown. Flip sides and cook the other side until brown.

Add some of the teriyaki sauce and mix well. Turn off the heat. Cool completely.

Place teriyaki seitan, squash and broccoli in meal prep containers. Store remaining teriyaki sauce in an airtight container. Place the containers in the refrigerator until use. It can last for 4 days.

Seitan and Mushrooms with Polenta

Ingredients:

For polenta:

- 4 cups vegetable broth or water

- Salt to taste

- Pepper to taste

- 1 ½ cups instant polenta

For mushroom and seitan:

- 4 tablespoons olive oil

- 4 tablespoons flour

- ½ cup white wine

- 2 teaspoons dried parsley

- 2 packages seitan (8 ounces each), cut into strips

- 16 ounces baby Portobello mushrooms, chopped

- 2 cups vegetable broth

- 2 tablespoons chopped fresh oregano

- 1 teaspoon garlic powder

- Salt to taste

- Pepper to taste

Serving day ingredients:

- ½ - 1 cup almond milk (optional)

Directions:

To make polenta: Add broth or water into the saucepan. Place the saucepan over medium heat. When it begins to simmer, add polenta and cook until nearly dry. Turn off the heat.

To make mushroom and seitan: Place a large skillet over medium heat. Add oil. When the oil is heated, add mushrooms and cook until slightly brown.

Add flour and stir for a few seconds. Stir in the wine and broth.

Stir in the herbs, salt and spices. Cook until thick.

Add seitan and cook for a couple of minutes. Turn off the heat and cool completely.

Transfer seitan and polenta into airtight containers and refrigerate until use. It can last for 3 days.

To serve: Add polenta into a pan. Add milk if using or some broth and heat the polenta.

Heat the mushrooms and seitan mixture.

Divide into bowls and serve.

Pho Soup

Ingredients:

- 2 cups very thinly sliced carrots

- 4 teaspoons minced fresh ginger

- 2 cups julienned red bell pepper

- 4 teaspoons minced garlic

- 4 cups uncooked, thin rice noodles

Serving day ingredients:

- 12 cups boiling hot vegetable stock

- 8 tablespoons soy sauce or tamari

Directions:

Take 4 wide-mouth Mason's jars. Divide all the ingredients into the jars, with noodles right on top.

Fasten the lid and refrigerate until use.

To serve: Add soy sauce and stock into the jars. Add some boiling water if the jar is not filled with the stock. Fasten the lid and set aside for 15 minutes.

Stir well. Season with salt and pepper to taste.

Baked Sheet Pan Ratatouille

Ingredients:

- 6 Japanese eggplants or 2 large eggplants, cut into ½ inch thick pieces

- 4 tomatoes, cut into ¾ inch thick wedges

- 2 onions, cut into ½ inch thick slices

- 1 red bell pepper, cut into ½ inch thick strips

- 1 yellow bell pepper, cut into ½ inch thick strips

- 24 – 28 whole garlic cloves, peeled

- 4 zucchinis or summer squash, halved lengthwise, cut into ½ inch thick slices crosswise

- 1 tablespoon fresh chopped thyme

- Salt to taste

- Pepper to taste

- Olive oil, as required

- Balsamic vinegar to taste

Serving options: Use any one

- Cooked pasta

- Cooked beans or whole grains

- Cooked polenta

- Toast

Directions:

Line 2 large baking sheets with parchment paper.

Place the vegetables on the baking sheets without overlapping. Place garlic cloves at different spots on the baking sheets.

Trickle some oil over the vegetables. Season with salt and pepper. Sprinkle thyme and mix using your hands.

Bake in a preheated oven at 400° F for about 30 minutes or until tender and slightly brown around the edges. Stir once halfway through baking.

Remove from the oven and transfer into an airtight container. Taste and adjust the seasoning if required. Sprinkle some vinegar and toss well.

Close the lid and refrigerate until use. It can last for 4 – 5 days. You can also transfer the roasted vegetables into freezer-safe bags. Freeze until use. It can last for 15 days.

To serve: Heat the vegetables in an oven. Serve with the suggested serving options.

Butternut Squash and Lentil Curry

Ingredients:

- 1 cup red lentils, rinsed

- ½ cup finely chopped onions

- 2 cups cubed butternut squash

- 1 tablespoon minced fresh ginger

- 1 large clove garlic, peeled, minced

- ½ tablespoon curry powder

- 1 teaspoon garam masala powder

- 1 teaspoon ground cumin

- 1 teaspoon ground coriander

- 1 teaspoon turmeric powder

- ½ can (from a 19 ounces can) diced tomatoes

- ½ can (from a 13.5 ounces can) coconut milk

- 1 ½ cups stock

- Salt to taste

- Lime juice to taste

Directions:

Add all the ingredients except lime juice into a soup pot.

Place the pot over medium heat. When it begins to boil, lower the heat and simmer until well cooked. Mash lightly if desired. Turn off the heat. Let it cool completely.

Add lime juice and stir. Transfer into an airtight container and refrigerate until use. It can last for 4 days. To freeze: Transfer into freezer bags and freeze until use. It can last for 3 months.

Avocado Fries (nuts)

INGREDIENTS:

1 tbsp. olive oil

½ cup almond flour

¼ tsp. cayenne pepper

¼ tsp. smoked paprika

Pinch of salt

¾ tbsp. unsweetened almond milk

1 medium Hass avocado (pitted, peeled)

1 tsp. lime juice

DIRECTIONS

Preheat the oven to 400°F/200°C.

Line a baking tray with parchment paper and grease the paper with the olive oil.

In a small bowl, combine the flour, cayenne pepper, smoked paprika, and salt.

Pour the almond milk into another small bowl.

Slice the peeled avocado into 10 equally-sized fries.

Coat all sides of the fries in the flour mixture, dip in almond milk, and coat with another layer of flour.

Transfer the coated fries to the greased baking tray.

Bake the fries for 5 minutes, then flip them over and bake for another 10 minutes. Flip the fries again and bake for 5 more minutes.

Flip the fries one more time, sprinkle them with the lime juice, and bake them for a final 5 minutes.

Take the baking tray out of the oven and allow the fries to cool down for a few minutes.

Serve warm with any low-carb (vegan) sauce and enjoy!

Alternatively, store the avocado fries in an airtight container in the fridge and consume within 2 days. Store in the freezer for a maximum of 30 days and thaw at room temperature. Reheat in the microwave for about 40-60 seconds.

Quick Veggie Protein Bowl (soy)

INGREDIENTS:

4 oz. extra-firm tofu (drained)

¼ tsp. turmeric

¼ tsp. cayenne pepper

1 tbsp. coconut oil

1 cup broccoli florets (diced)

1 cup Chinese kale (diced)

½ cup button mushrooms (diced)

½ tsp. dried oregano

Himalayan salt and ground black pepper to taste

½ tsp. paprika

Optional: ¼ cup of fresh oregano (diced)

DIRECTIONS

Cut the tofu into tiny pieces and season with the turmeric and cayenne pepper.

Warm a large skillet over medium heat and add ¾ of the coconut oil.

Once oil is heated, add the tofu and cook it for about 5 minutes, stirring continuously.

Transfer the cooked tofu to a medium-sized bowl and set it aside.

Add the remaining coconut oil, diced broccoli florets, Chinese kale, button mushrooms, and the remaining herbs to the skillet. Season with the salt, pepper, and paprika to taste.

Cook the vegetables for 6-8 minutes, stirring continuously.

Turn off the heat and transfer the cooked veggies and tofu to the bowl. Garnish with the optional fresh oregano.

Serve and enjoy!

Alternatively, store the quick veggie protein bowl in an airtight container in the fridge and consume within 4 days. Store for a maximum of 60 days in the freezer and thaw at room temperature before serving.

Special Zucchini Lasagna (soy, nuts)

INGREDIENTS:

Walnut Sauce:

1 cup walnuts (ground)

1 cup simple marinara sauce (*see recipe*)

¼ cup sundried tomatoes (chopped)

Optional: pinch of salt

Tofu Ricotta:

1 14-oz. package firm tofu (drained)

¼ cup fresh basil

1 tbsp. lemon juice

4 tbsp. nutritional yeast

2 small garlic cloves (minced)

1½ tbsp. olive oil

Salt and pepper to taste

Lasagna:

2 zucchinis (thinly sliced)

2 cups simple marinara sauce (*see recipe*)

Salt and pepper to taste

DIRECTIONS

Preheat the oven to 375°F/190°C.

Add the walnut sauce ingredients to a blender. Blend the ingredients into an almost completely smooth mixture.

Transfer the mixture to a medium-sized bowl and set it aside.

Clean the blender container and then add all tofu ricotta ingredients. Blend until smooth.

Take a large loaf pan and add 2 cups of simple marinara sauce. Cover the sauce with the zucchini slices and top these with ⅓ of the tofu ricotta. Pour half of the walnut sauce on top.

Make another layer, starting with zucchini slices, then tofu ricotta, and then the remaining walnut sauce.

Finish the lasagna with a layer of zucchini slices and tofu ricotta. Top the dish with some additional salt and pepper to taste.

Transfer the lasagna to the oven and bake for 30-35 minutes.

Allow the lasagna to cool down before serving and enjoy!

Baked Cajun salmon

Ingredients:

Four salmon fillets

½ onion, sliced

2 peppers, yellow and red, in stripes

3 garlic cloves, pressed

Sea salt and pepper to taste

3 tbsp olive oil, native

1 tsp thyme, dried

1 tsp Cajun spice

2 teaspoons paprika powder

2 teaspoons of garlic powder

Directions

Preheat oven to 200 degrees and lay out a baking tray with parchment paper.

Put the onions, peppers and garlic on the baking sheet. Season with salt and pepper and drizzle with a little olive oil.

Put the thyme, Cajun spice, paprika, and garlic powder in a bowl and mix together.

Also, lay salmon fillets on baking sheet and cover with the spice mixture.

Bake vegetables and salmon for about 20-25 minutes.

Remove salmon and vegetables from the oven and serve warm.

Chapter 14: Dessert Recipes

Blueberry Lemon Choco Cups

INGREDIENTS:

½ cup cocoa butter

½ cup coconut oil

¼ cup cocoa powder

2 tbsp. organic lemon zest

¼ cup fresh lemon juice

½ tsp. stevia powder

20 blueberries

DIRECTIONS

Put the cocoa butter and coconut oil in a medium-sized bowl. Heat this bowl in the microwave for 10 seconds, until the butter and oil have melted. Make sure it doesn't get too hot.

Take the bowl out of the microwave and mix in all the remaining ingredients. Make sure everything is well incorporated.

Line a muffin tray with muffin liners.

Scoop the soft mixture out of the bowl with a tablespoon into the muffin liners. If the mixture isn't soft enough to be transferred, heat it again in the microwave for 10 seconds.

Fill all the muffin liners evenly, 1 tablespoon at a time.

Refrigerate the cups for 45 minutes, until the choco cups are firm. Take the cups out, serve and enjoy!

Alternatively, store the blueberry lemon cups in the fridge, within 6 days. Store at room temperature

Peanut Butter Power Bars (peanuts, nuts)

INGREDIENTS:

¼ cup almond butter

½ cup peanut butter (*see recipe*)

½ cup coconut oil

¼ cup sunflower seeds

¼ cup walnuts (chopped)

¼ cup hemp seeds

1 tbsp. vanilla extract

1 tsp. stevia powder

DIRECTIONS

Put the almond butter, peanut butter, and coconut oil in a small saucepan. Heat the saucepan over medium-low heat and whisk the ingredients until everything is molten and fully incorporated.

Take the saucepan off the heat and set the mixture aside to cool down.

Line a baking dish with parchment paper.

Pour the contents of the saucepan into a medium-sized bowl and mix in the remaining ingredients.

Transfer the mixture onto the baking dish and spread it out into an even layer.

Put the baking dish in the freezer for 45 minutes, until the chunk is firm.

Take the baking dish out the freezer and cut the chunk into the desired number of bars.

Dark Chocolate Mint Cups (nuts)

INGREDIENTS:

½ cup cocoa butter

½ cup almond butter

¼ cup coconut oil

¼ cup cocoa powder (unsweetened)

1 tsp. mint extract

1 tbsp. vanilla extract

1 tsp. stevia powder

DIRECTIONS

Put the cocoa butter, almond butter, and coconut oil in a small saucepan. Heat the pan over medium-low heat. Incorporate the ingredients using a whisk, add the cocoa powder, and whisk again until all ingredients are fully incorporated.

Take the saucepan off the heat and set it aside to cool down.

Line a baking dish with parchment paper.

Pour the mixture from the saucepan into a medium-sized bowl and mix in all the remaining ingredients. Make sure all ingredients are fully incorporated.

Transfer a tablespoon of the mixture from the bowl into each muffin liner.

Repeat this process until the bowl is empty, making sure that all 16 muffin liners are evenly filled.

Refrigerate the cups for 45 minutes, until the coconut cups are firm.

Take the cups out of the freezer, serve, and enjoy right away.

Alternatively, store the chocolate mint cups in the fridge, within 6 days. Store at room temperature

Espresso Protein Cups (soy, nuts)

INGREDIENTS:

1 cup almond butter (or cashew butter)

¼ cup coconut oil

¼ cup organic soy protein (chocolate flavor)

2 tsp. instant espresso powder (or instant coffee powder)

½ tsp. stevia powder

Optional: 1 tbsp. full-fat coconut milk

DIRECTIONS

Line a cupcake tin with nine cupcake liners and set it aside.

Heat a medium-sized saucepan over medium-low heat and add all the ingredients, including the optional coconut milk.

Incorporate all ingredients while stirring constantly. If desired, add more espresso powder, stevia powder, coconut milk, and/or soy protein to taste.

Divide the mixture equally into the nine cupcake liners and transfer the tin to the freezer.

After 30 minutes, take the cupcake tin out, serve the cups and enjoy!

Alternatively, store the espresso protein cups in the fridge using an airtight container and consume within 7 days.

Tip: This makes a perfect ketogenic snack to start the day with, thanks to the natural caffeine from coffee!

3-Ingredient Berry Bites

INGREDIENTS:

1 cup coconut oil

½ cup mixed berries (fresh or frozen)

1 tsp. vanilla extract

DIRECTIONS

Line a baking tray with parchment paper and set it aside.

Heat a medium-sized saucepan over medium-low heat and add the coconut oil.

Once the oil has melted, take the saucepan off the heat and transfer its contents to a food processor or blender.

Add the berries and the vanilla extract and process until all ingredients are incorporated and smooth.

Spread the mixture into a square form on the baking tray.

Transfer the baking tray to the freezer and allow the chunk to set. This should take about 25 minutes.

Take out the baking tray, remove the chunk, and cut it into 6 equal pieces.

Serve the berry bites and enjoy!

Alternatively, store the bites in the fridge using an airtight container and consume within 4 days.

Coconut Chia Pudding

Ingredients:

4 cups coconut milk, unsweetened

3 tablespoons agave nectar

1 cup chia seeds

1 large mango, peeled, pitted, chopped

Directions

Add milk, agave nectar, and chia seeds to a bowl and stir. Transfer into individual dessert bowls.

Chill for 5-6 hours.

Top with mango and serve.

Plum Protein Parfait

Ingredients:

For the plum layer:

4 cups plums, pitted, chopped

2 tablespoons maple syrup

1 teaspoon vanilla extract

For the coconut cream layer:

1/2 cup coconut milk

2 small bananas, sliced, frozen

For the chia pudding layer:

8 tablespoons chia seeds

2 tablespoons ground cinnamon

2 cups soy milk or almond milk

4 tablespoons maple syrup

2 teaspoons ground ginger

For the crumble layer:

1 cup whole wheat flour

2 cups oats

1/2 cup almond milk or soy milk

8 Medjool dates, pitted

4 tablespoons coconut oil, melted

6 tablespoons shredded coconut, unsweetened

Directions

To make crumble layer: Mix oats and flour together in a bowl.

Blend together the rest of the ingredients of the crumble layer until smooth. Add this mixture into the bowl of oats and stir.

Transfer the ingredients to a greased baking dish.

Bake in a preheated oven at 400° F for about 15 minutes or until golden brown on top.

Remove from the oven. When cool enough to handle, crumble it and bake until crunchy.

To make plum layer: Mix together plum, maple syrup, and vanilla and set aside.

To make chia pudding layer: Add all the ingredients of this layer to a bowl and stir and set aside.

To make coconut cream layer: Add coconut milk and banana slices to a blender and blend until smooth.

To assemble: Take 6 glasses or masons jars. Divide and spoon in the plum mixture to make the bottom layer.

Next layer with coconut cream layer, followed by the chia pudding layer, and finally top with the crumble layer.

Chill and serve.

Chocó-Berry Cheese Cake

Ingredients:

For the crust:

1 1/2 cups porridge oats

6 tablespoons almond milk

1/2 teaspoon cocoa powder

A large pinch salt

For the cream layer:

4 cups cannellini beans

½ cup almond milk

4 teaspoons stevia or any sweetener of your choice

2 scoops pea protein powder

1 teaspoon vanilla extract

For the chocolate layer:

1 tablespoon cocoa powder

2 teaspoons stevia

2 tablespoons almond milk

For the berry layer:

1 cup berries

2 teaspoons stevia

1 scoop pea protein powder

Directions

To make the crust: Mix together all of the ingredients for the crust. Transfer into a cake tin. Press well.

To make the cream layer: Add the cannellini beans, almond milk, stevia, pea protein powder, and vanilla to a food processor. Pulse until well combined. Remove from the food processor and take out about a cup of the mixture and keep in a bowl. To this, add the chocolate layer ingredients.

Spread this chocolate layer over the prepared crust.

To the remaining beans mixture, add berries and sweetener to it. Blend until smooth.

Spread over the chocolate layer.

Garnish with berries and sprinkle the coconut flakes.

Refrigerate until well chilled. Chop into wedges and serve.

Easy Chocó-Nut Ice cream

Ingredients:

6 bananas, sliced, frozen

1/2 cup creamy peanut butter

1/2 cup unsweetened cocoa powder

3 teaspoons vanilla extract

Agave nectar or sweetener of your choice to taste

Directions

Blend together all the ingredients in a blender until smooth. Transfer into a bowl. Using a hand mixer, beat it until fluffy.

Pour the mixture into a freezer-safe container and freeze until done.

Dragon Fruit Pudding

Ingredients:

For the pudding:

7 ounces of frozen dragon fruit puree

2 cups frozen chopped mango

1 kiwi, peeled, chopped

2 cups frozen pineapple

2 cups baby spinach

1 cup almond milk or soy milk, unsweetened

4 tablespoons agave nectar

4 scoops vanilla pea protein powder

For the topping:

1/2 cup blackberries

1/2 cup blueberries

1 banana, sliced

4 tablespoons pumpkin seeds

4 tablespoons almonds, chopped

4 teaspoons chia seeds

Directions

Add all the ingredients of the pudding to a blender and blend until smooth.

Transfer into dessert bowls. Chill for an hour.

Meanwhile toast the almonds and pumpkin seeds.

Remove from the refrigerator. Top with blackberries, blueberries, banana, almonds, pumpkin seeds, and chia seeds.

Serve immediately.

Puffed Quinoa Peanut Butter Balls

Ingredients:

2 cups puffed quinoa

1 cup peanut butter

1/2 cup agave nectar

2 tablespoons crushed peanuts

2 teaspoons vanilla extract

Dairy-free dark chocolate, melted (optional)

Directions

Mix together in a heatproof bowl, peanut butter, agave, and vanilla. Place the bowl in a double boiler for a while until the ingredients are softened and smooth flowing.

Remove from heat and add puffed quinoa. Mix well and refrigerate for 15-20 minutes.

Remove from the refrigerator and form small balls. Dip into dark chocolate if desired. Refrigerate again for 15 minutes before serving.

Matcha Coconut Balls

INGREDIENTS:

1 cup coconut oil

1 cup coconut butter

½ cup full-fat coconut milk (refrigerated)

1 ½ tsp. matcha green tea powder

1 tsp. vanilla extract

2 tbsp. organic lemon zest

Pinch of sea salt

1 cup shredded coconut

DIRECTIONS

Add all the ingredients except the shredded coconut to a medium-sized bowl. Microwave the bowl for a few seconds until the coconut oil has melted.

Use a mixer to combine all ingredients in the bowl.

Cover the bowl and transfer it to the refrigerator.

Line a baking tray with parchment paper and spread the shredded coconut over it.

After one hour, take the bowl out of the fridge and use a tablespoon to form 16 balls.

Coat each ball in the shredded coconut and line them up on a baking tray.

Transfer the tray into the fridge for another 15 minutes.

Serve the matcha coconut balls and enjoy!

Alternatively, store the balls in the fridge using an airtight container and consume within 12 days.

Tip: Can't get enough of the matcha? Coat the balls in both the shredded coconut and some additional matcha green tea powder

Red Velvet Protein Bites

Ingredients:

1/2 cup almond meal or almond flour

6 tablespoons coconut flour

2 teaspoons beetroot powder

6 tablespoons plant-based vanilla protein powder

4 tablespoons cocoa powder

3/4 cup dairy-free dark chocolate

6 tablespoons almond milk

2 teaspoons vanilla extract

2 tablespoons coconut oil, melted

Directions

Mix together in a bowl, almond meal, coconut flour, beetroot powder, and protein powder.

Add rest of the ingredients and mix well.

Transfer onto a lined baking sheet and spread well with a rolling pin.

Freeze for 15 minutes.

Meanwhile, melt dark chocolate in a microwave.

Remove the baking sheet from the freezer and chop into squares. Dip the squares into the melted chocolate and place it back on the baking sheet.

Chill again and serve.

Cheesecake Cups (soy, nuts)

INGREDIENTS:

Crust:

½ cup pumpkin seeds (raw)

6 tbsp. shredded coconut (unsweetened)

3 tbsp. coconut oil

2 tbsp. organic soy protein (vanilla flavor)

½ tsp. stevia powder

Pinch of salt

Filling:

6 tbsp. coconut oil

6 tbsp. almond butter

6 tbsp. coconut cream

2 tbsp. lemon juice

2 tbsp. organic soy protein (vanilla flavor)

Pinch of salt

Optional: ¼ tsp. xanthan gum

Optional: ¼ tsp. stevia powder (or more to taste)

DIRECTIONS

Line a cupcake tin with 6 cupcake liners.

Heat a small frying pan over medium-high heat.

Toast the pumpkin seeds in the frying pan, stirring occasionally for about 4 minutes.

Add the shredded coconut and stir thoroughly to toast everything evenly.

Take the frying pan off the heat and allow the ingredients to cool down before transferring them into a food processor or blender. Pulse the pumpkin seeds and shredded coconut into small crumbs.

Transfer the crumbs to a medium-sized bowl and add the remaining crust ingredients.

Combine all ingredients into a thick dough and divide this mixture into six equal-sized balls.

Put one ball into each of the cupcake liners, pressing and flattening the balls into a crust at the bottom of each cupcake liner.

Transfer the tin into the freezer and prepare the filling.

Heat a medium-sized saucepan over medium heat and add the coconut oil. Remove the saucepan from the heat once the coconut oil has melted.

Put the melted coconut oil, almond butter, coconut cream, lemon juice, organic soy protein, and a pinch of salt to the (uncleaned) food processor or blender. Process these ingredients until well combined with a smooth and creamy texture.

Add the optional xanthan gum and stevia. Xanthan gum will help thicken the cheesecake fat bombs, while the stevia will add a sweeter flavor. Use slightly more or less stevia to taste.

Take the cupcake tin out of the freezer and top all crusts with filling. Make sure to divide the filling equally among the 6 cups with a tablespoon.

Transfer the tin back into the fridge until the cups are firm.

Serve the cheesecake cups at room temperature and enjoy!

Alternatively, store the cups in the fridge inside an airtight container and consume within 5 days.

Green Tea & Ginger Cups (nuts)

INGREDIENTS:

1 cup coconut oil

2 tbsp. almond butter

2-inch piece of ginger (finely grated)

1 tbsp. low-carb maple syrup

4 tbsp. matcha green tea powder

Pinch of Himalayan salt

Optional: ½ tsp. stevia powder

DIRECTIONS

Line a cupcake tin with six cupcake papers and set it aside.

Heat a medium-sized saucepan over low heat and add the coconut oil.

Once the coconut oil has become soft and spreadable, remove the saucepan from the heat and transfer the oil to a medium-sized bowl.

Add the remaining ingredients and stir until all ingredients are combined and no lumps remain. Blend in the optional stevia powder if you prefer a sweeter flavor. Use slightly more or less stevia to taste.

Divide the mixture among the six cupcake papers and transfer the tin to the freezer.

After 30 minutes, take the cupcake tin out, serve and enjoy!

Alternatively, store the green tea cups in the fridge using an airtight container and consume within 5 days.

No-Carb Cereal Bars (nuts)

INGREDIENTS:

1 cup pumpkin seeds

1 cup sunflower seeds

1 cup almonds

1 cup hazelnuts (chopped)

1 flax egg (*see recipe*)

¼ cup almond butter

¼ cup cocoa butter

1 tsp. stevia powder

Ground cinnamon to taste

DIRECTIONS

Preheat oven to 350°F/175°C, and line a shallow baking dish with parchment paper.

Transfer all the listed ingredients to a blender or food processor. Blend it into a chunky mixture.

Transfer the mixture onto the baking dish and spread it out evenly into a flat chunk on the parchment paper.

Bake this chunk for about 15 minutes.

Take the baking dish out of the oven and let cool down for about 10 minutes.

Cut the chunk into the desired number of bars while it's still a bit warm.

CONCLUSION

Whether you've already begun your journey as a vegan or are just starting to implicate an animal-product-free diet, veganism is one of the best jumping-off points when you are beginning a new fitness regime. Especially if you've decided to eat on a Ketogenic diet plan, a vegan diet allows you to begin your Keto journey from a healthier and more body-conscious state of mind. However, there are a few pointers to cover before you begin eating a low-carb, high-fat Keto diet to make sure that you're eating the healthiest possible vegan options already. The Keto diet is notoriously restrictive when it comes to food choices, and so it can be a bit tricky for someone whose eating habits are already quite limited to further shrink their pool of options. The bright side is that your options are limited in a great way! Implicating a Ketogenic diet on top of your vegan lifestyle means that you're starting with a toolbox half-full of healthy habits that will maximize your Keto success.

If you haven't already been tracking your "macros and micros" for your regular vegan diet, it's about time that you started. There is no better way to make sure you're getting the exact amount of calories, and the exact amount of nutrients, that your body needs without tracking your macros and micros. "Macros" is an abbreviation that stands for "macronutrients," and they're what the Keto diet is based on. The three main macronutrients required for human life are carbohydrates, proteins, and fats. That's right! Tracking your macronutrients is just as easy as tracking how many grams of protein, carbohydrates, and fats you're eating in each meal.

Best of Luck!